st great relationships don't start with a bang. In this excel-
book, you will learn how to get off that emotional roller
ster before it ruins your life."

—Scott Barry Kaufman, PhD, psychologist,
author, and host of *The Psychology Podcast*

pe-igniting, shame-eradicating . . . *Why Do We Stay?* pro-
s absolution from the suffering many of us endure in silence,
lated by guilt and isolation. An empathy- and informa-
-rich resource that gives voice to the voiceless, this book is
mming with heart-expanding vulnerability, healing insights,
radical honesty."

—Kirbee Miller, author and speaker

Why Do We Stay? Stephanie grieves many things—a roman-
relationship, the dream of what could have been, and the
s she lost in that relationship. We all have a personal jour-
with grief. This book outlines Stephanie's journey through
, which informed how she grieved, and which ultimately
ught her back to herself."

—Kimberly Goessele, former CEO of Alive Hospice

WHY DO WE STAY?

How My Toxic Relationship Can Help You Find Freedom

STEPHANIE QUAYLE

WITH W. KEITH CAMPBELL, PHD

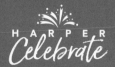

Why Do We Stay?

Published by Harper Celebrate, an imprint of HarperCollins Focus LLC.

Note: The information in this book has been carefully researched by the authors, and is intended to be a source of information only. Readers are urged to consult with their physicians or other advisors to address specific medical issues. The authors and the publisher assume no responsibility for any injuries suffered or damages or losses incurred during or as a result of the use or application of the information contained herein.

Names and identifying characteristics of some individuals have been changed to preserve their privacy.

Any internet addresses (websites, blogs, etc.) in this book are offered as a resource. They are not intended in any way to be or imply an endorsement by HarperCollins Focus LLC, nor does HarperCollins Focus LLC vouch for the content of these sites for the life of this book.

Photography credits for book jacket: John Shearer (top) and Jason Thrasher (bottom).

Cover design: Milkglass Creative

Song lyrics by Stephanie Quayle, courtesy of Big Sky Music Group.

ISBN 978-1-4002-4453-9 (audiobook)
ISBN 978-1-4002-4452-2 (eBook)
ISBN 978-1-4002-4451-5 (HC)

Printed in Malaysia

24 25 26 27 28 SEM 5 4 3 2 1

David, if this had never happened,
we would never have happened.
Thank you for your love and patience.

Pull up a seat and have yourself a listen
Let's start at the end to get to the beginning
Hell, I wouldn't believe it if I didn't live it
Sometimes the truth is stranger than fiction

—STEPHANIE QUAYLE,
FROM HER SONG "FICTION"

CONTENTS

24 *hours before . . .*

I tell him to call the airport so they can get his plane ready. "Let's fly to Vegas. I feel lucky," I say with unrelenting enthusiasm.

He's taken by my newfound spontaneity. I was never the spontaneous one, but he was all in. I felt like the luckiest girl alive.

A few hours later . . .

We can't fly out because a storm's coming—thunderstorms, lightning, ominous skies—as if the weather knows something I don't.

We head home, spend an amazing night together. Our love drowns out the storms.

The next morning . . .

The romance of yesterday is traded for a dismissive coolness.

My friend Michelle comes over and asks why I stay. She listens as I explain he's not always like that. When he's good, he's great.

She tells me I'll never leave him.

That evening . . .

 I'm in the kitchen making dinner when I get a call. *The* call. The one you don't want.

 "There's been an accident. You better come quickly."

 But I didn't get there in time. He was gone.

Michelle was right. I wouldn't leave him. I *didn't* leave him.

 He died.

 That's how I got out of my toxic relationship.

INTRODUCTION

I didn't leave my first toxic relationship.

I stayed.

But the simple fact that it ended didn't mean I was well or healed or ready for another relationship. I wasn't. In fact, when I began dating again, I ended up in another toxic relationship.

I know what it's like to be in the trenches. I'm familiar with what it feels like to be shamed, blamed, minimized, disrespected, love bombed, and gaslighted. As someone who was in a toxic relationship for years, I know what it feels like to silence my voice so as not to make waves. I know how to make myself small in a relationship so the other person has plenty of room to feel big. I know what it is to question my own perceptions of reality, never really trusting myself or my intuition. I know what it is to dismiss and ignore the concerns of family and friends who love me—to believe desperately that it wasn't as bad as it really was.

But you know what? It *was* bad.

I couldn't have written this book a dozen years ago, or even *two* years ago. It has taken me fourteen years since the death of my toxic partner, Paulo, before I could share my story with you.

Ultimately, though, this book isn't about me. It's about *you*.

In these pages, I'm welcoming you into my story in the hopes that you might catch some glimpses of your own—or of someone you care about. Chapter by chapter, we'll walk through the relationship I *didn't* leave, the one I *did* leave, and—if you stick with me—eventually to the one I'll *never* leave. (Trust me, it's worth sticking around.)

And there's the win, right? Just because we've been stuck in something that was unhealthy doesn't mean we weren't made for something better. It doesn't mean we don't deserve something better. We do. I do. *You* do. But in order to be ready for something better, we need to do the good rigorous work of healing so that we're ready when it comes along.

As a country music recording artist, I'm a storyteller. I'm

here for it. Bad relationships? They are country music *gold*. But believe me when I tell you that my story is one I never would have chosen to tell. Nor is it one I would have chosen to *live*. Although it took me a minute—7,358,500 minutes to be exact— I've done the work. I've found my freedom. I'm living well. I'm not telling this story today for me. The only reason I believe my story is worth telling is because of you.

If I found freedom from my past, you can too.

You can get your time back, your years back. You can begin to use your voice again. You can learn to trust your gut again. You can become the vibrant, robust person you were made to be. You can be honest and transparent about your relationships with the people who care about you. By rejecting toxic relationships, you can choose to *live well*.

In each chapter I'll show you a glimpse of my story on this journey to freedom. And along the way, at critical and relevant points in my story, you're going to hear from Dr. W. Keith Campbell, a professor at the University of Georgia's Department of Psychology. Dr. Campbell will shine a light on the yellow flags—and red ones!—I missed so that you can learn to spot them in your own relationships and not lose any more time. I lost years being in and grieving toxic relationships, but you don't have to.

Dr. Campbell will also define some of the language in this conversation about toxic relationships. For instance:

> **TOXIC RELATIONSHIP:** a relationship between two people who don't relate to each other in healthy ways. A relationship with more conflict than is typical or necessary. A relationship in which one person exploits, distorts, or minimizes the perspective and experience of the other person. In this kind of relationship, neither partner is growing or flourishing. Instead, you see hostility, anxiety, uncertainty, victimization, and abuse.

At the end of each chapter, Dr. Campbell will offer some questions for you to reflect on as a way to connect some of these new ideas to your own life, or as you consider your relationship with someone you love.

Sharing my story with you is another step in my healing journey that continues every day. It's not over. My hope and prayer is that *Why Do We Stay?* will empower you to take the next step in your journey toward freedom.

You are stronger than you think. You are stronger than you know. You are your greatest advocate.

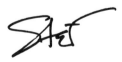

WHEN YOU'RE IN A TOXIC RELATIONSHIP

didn't know I was in a toxic relationship when I was in it. Who does? It's so much easier in hindsight to see things clearly, to see a relationship for what it was. It's been fourteen years and only now can I see it clearly and understand the relationship dynamics fully.

Maybe you're where I was fourteen years ago, trapped in something that doesn't make sense or confused by your relationship. Maybe it's not toxic but it's certainly not healthy. Maybe you are just starting to see cracks or warning signs and are wondering what the foundation of this relationship is—and whether you should stay or go.

I can't tell you what to do or how to react. But I can walk you through the phases of my relationship and my path toward freedom and healing afterward—and maybe you'll learn or receive something that helps you make sense of your own situation. That's my hope.

Why do *we* stay? It's plural for a reason. There's a *we* here. You are not alone. I am not alone. We are here for each other.

1

LIFE WAS PERFECT

---

*The Lies We Believe When
We're Sold a Dream*

When your relationship starts off like a fairy tale, with all the signs of promise and passion that will lead to a happily ever after, you're not thinking of much else—let alone all the ways it could go wrong. And why should you?

Not all relationships that start off this way end badly. I didn't know mine was ending badly until after it was over. But there were a few lies in the beginning that I was willing to believe and happily bought into.

LIE #1: BEAUTIFUL BEGINNINGS ALWAYS STAY THAT WAY

When I met Paulo for the first time, it caught me off guard because I wasn't looking for him.

The Santa Monica ocean breeze danced its way up to Fourteenth and Montana, where Planet Blue, a high-end, beachy, boho-chic clothing boutique, was *the* place—the place in Los Angeles where people from all around the world would come to get a glimpse of celebrity and the latest wearable style by long-haired California dreamers. A mix of Malibu and street chic and your best friend's closet. It was a place the locals had made the community hub for dressing-room confessions and last-minute finds for that TV appearance or star-studded gala.

On a sleepy December evening, I was closing up the shop after a long day at work. I had already sent everyone else home and was about to reconcile the day when I felt eyes on me through the massive floor-to-ceiling glass door. I looked up to see who wanted to shop after hours, and then our eyes met. His light ocean eyes immediately pulled me in. He stood there with his daughter, her eyes the same greenish hue. He was desperate to find a small gift for a birthday party for which they were running late. How could I stand in the way of a father trying so hard to make his little girl's night perfect?

I helped them find the perfect gift, and in that moment, I was the hero to this dad, and he got to be her hero. I had flyers by the register for my upcoming full-band show the following Tuesday. So, like any shameless, self-promoting artist, I enthusiastically shared about my show and handed him a flyer. He said he'd try to make it and would bring a friend. He then introduced himself as Paulo, and the quiet girl studying my every move was his daughter, Eden.

It wasn't just Paulo who got my attention that first day. I was so taken by Eden; she grabbed ahold of my heart the moment I looked down at her curious eyes, tanned skin, and sun-kissed hair. She embodied a song without even trying. She was a song all on her own.

My relationship with Paulo developed slowly, in stages, the way you would expect a trusted relationship to go. After my show at a place called The Gig in Hollywood, Paulo hired me to teach Eden guitar over the next few years, a role that grew into being a nanny to Eden—and friend, confidante. Eventually, he would introduce me to his friends as his "little sis."

As more time passed, I went from being introduced as Paulo's little sister to engaging in public displays of affection. From words of friendship to him wanting me as his one and only. And I fell for him—"Hook, line, and sinker, like a trout in the Yellowstone."[1] He was larger than life, and I was now a part of his life.

Feelings between us had changed. The moment he held my face in his weathered hands, it was over. His muscular build fused with my small frame, and it felt like we were never going to let go. I had never known this kind of love could exist. It was passionate, adventurous, a meet-you-where-you-are, grown-up kind of love.

Every day was a new experience, and the word *no* never crossed my lips. If "floating on a cloud" describes a girl in love, that was me. There was nothing I wouldn't do for Paulo. His intensity for living was unlike anything I had ever experienced. His gaze felt intoxicating. If he was a storm, I was dancing in the rain. If he was the hurricane, I was in the eye of it. I was young, in love, and sure of it all. How could it go wrong?

Toxic in Disguise: Too Good to Be True

Relationships can start off as amazing and exciting but then transition to something negative over time. Toxic, controlling, and dishonest people aren't attractive as relationship partners, so it shouldn't be too surprising that these people will often hide those toxic traits and instead put on a positive front when you first meet them.

In the initial stages of attraction, you might have a partner who is charming, has high status, and is attractive.

They appear to be very interested in you, which can be intoxicating. When this interest becomes extreme, it's called "love bombing."

LOVE BOMBING: a large amount of positive attention and praise given to a potential romantic partner who is overwhelmed by the affection and falls under the spell of the love bomber. After commitment is established, the love bombing diminishes and is replaced with efforts to control.

As relationships move toward emotional intimacy and commitment, from something fun and exciting to something more serious, we naturally desire and expect trust, loyalty, and love. But with toxic partners, instead of a deep emotional commitment, you get dishonesty, game-playing, infidelity, and physical and/or emotional abuse. Eventually, the relationship with the toxic partner collapses under its own weight, and you are stuck wondering why you were so attracted to that person in the first place.

Here is the reality: We are often attracted to people who are confident, charismatic, charming, and who flatter us. This is totally normal. Some individuals with these traits are authentic, but others will take advantage of us. It's impossible to know just from meeting someone which way the relationship is going to go. My suggestion is to always look at the potential partner's track record in relationships. Toxic individuals will leave a trail of wreckage behind them, much like a tornado moving through a town. If you find yourself starting a relationship with someone like this, consider a different partner. People are generally consistent, and you are likely to experience the same negativity that the last partner experienced.

—Dr. W. Keith Campbell

Note: all future shaded sections are by Dr. Campbell

LIE #2: I COULD HAVE IT ALL

Part of the dream I bought into with Paulo was the sense that I could have everything I always wanted: the guy, the home, the career, the family—the whole package.

We dreamed of building a home together. Paulo lived in an airplane hangar at the Santa Monica Airport. Nothing about the converted hangar was legal, but it suited Paulo, who liked to play by his own rules. Paulo also owned a little piece of land in Malibu we called "our place," where we would one day build the home that would house our love. Until then, our Airstream would be where we dreamed, played guitars, and shared starry nights, questioning nothing and living only for the moment.

My heart was unrestricted, and I hung on every word that came out of that mouth with the crooked smile. We eventually hired an architect and started planning our home. All was falling into place.

> My heart was unrestricted, and I hung on every word that came out of that mouth with the crooked smile.

One of the biggest allures of my relationship with Paulo was the chance to be a part of Eden's life and part of a family. I came from a broken family; my parents split when I was three and my brother was six. We endured the "back-and-forth, who gets who, split holidays, kids in the middle" divorced family model. Growing up, I had pretended to be a mommy many times with my dolls and my brother's G.I. Joes before my little half brothers came along. Not to mention I always mothered my big brother to a fault.

When I was sixteen, I signed myself up for a foreign exchange program in Switzerland, a place known for peace and neutrality.

The forms asked, "What kind of family do you want to pair with?" and I remember so badly wanting the nuclear family: mom, dad, and kids all living under one roof. In other words, not divorced. Even then, I wanted the perfect family: unbroken, unmessy.

When Eden came into my life, my dream of the perfect family grew even more. I naturally took on a lot of maternal roles, from school pickups to errands to all the rest. I became integral to our little family. I could calm Paulo when he got frustrated with Eden or her mom, and could lessen the blowback so Eden didn't bear the brunt of her parents' mutual contempt. I wasn't there to replace her mom or get in anyone's way. I was just a young woman in love trying to help a little girl navigate this complicated world with her parents. After all, it was a world I understood.

Over and over, Paulo would tell me what a good mother figure I was and how he was going to give us all we ever wanted in a family. I could have it all, or so I thought. On the hard days, if I ever thought about ending things with him or leaving, I would think of Eden and how I needed to be there for her. I was her family, and she was mine. She was as close to a child of my own as I had ever known. And when I pulled away, Paulo would double down on his love for me and reiterate his desire to build a family together.

Staying Committed to a Toxic Relationship

It doesn't always make sense to us why people stick with relationships that from the outside appear toxic, or at least very unhappy. We should only stay in relationships with people who love us and have our best interests at heart. But reality is often more complicated than that. If you're a teenager in a dating relationship, it can be easy to leave. When you're in a relationship as a mature adult, leaving the relationship isn't that easy for many reasons: time and emotional work invested, not to mention shared investments, such as a house or children.

All marriages have ups and downs, so making it hard to leave isn't necessarily a bad thing. But when you're with a toxic partner and in a dangerous, abusive relationship, these commitments can sometimes make you feel imprisoned.

If you find yourself overly invested or committed in a relationship that might not be going well, start investing outside of the relationship. Develop friendships, find a way to earn money or save money, or do other things so that your decision to stay in the relationship is based on what is healthy for you. Remember, it's your choice to stay, and you can always make the choice to leave, even if it feels impossible in the moment. You don't want to be forced to stay in a toxic or abusive relationship because you are trapped financially or socially. At the extremes, there are places like battered women's shelters, which offer an alternative for women who feel trapped in a toxic relationship they can't financially afford to escape.

LIE #3: I WAS SPECIAL AND UNIQUE

When Paulo and I first met, he wasn't interested in me as anything more than a friend—a pal. In fact, I had a boyfriend at the time, and it never even dawned on me that there would or could be more between us. Paulo would often bring me along on his dates so I could babysit Eden.

It was platonic. And then . . . it wasn't.

If you've come from a broken home or have experienced rocky roads with guys like I have, when a "nice" one comes along and tells you that you're special and they've never met anyone like you, it goes to the core of your being.

When our relationship turned romantic, Paulo made

me feel like I was the only woman—the only *person*—in the world at times, and it fed my desire to be loved and wanted and seen.

The way he trusted me to take care of Eden—from the guitar lessons and school pickups to everything else—confirmed that he accepted me in a way so different from anyone else. He was older and knew me in a way that felt so easy. Even though Paulo loved to make everyone laugh and was always the center of attention, I didn't get lost in his shadow.

My coworkers at Planet Blue watched our whole love story unfold. He would show up spontaneously with a handful of fresh-cut lilies. I had never liked lilies since they'd always symbolized death to me—funeral flowers. And yet I learned to love them as I loved Paulo. We lived as if no one else existed—or maybe we believed everyone was watching us.

Anytime he wanted to fly his plane and kiss the skies, I jumped at the chance, never considering the dangers of getting in an airplane with him. I trusted him with everything in me. From the aerial dogfights over the Malibu skies to the little stops at a small airport in Camarillo where we would grab a cheeseburger with the guys, flying felt so freeing. I thought maybe one day I would learn to fly too.

I knew we were getting serious when he brought me down to his hometown of Lafayette, Louisiana, where his family gathered. In moments like this, I felt we were the family I wanted us to be. He walked with pride, enjoying how impressed his Louisiana crew was by his domesticated ways and this young blonde on his arm.

Feeling Like a Trophy

Narcissistic men often look at their relationship partners like trophies or conquests. We use the term "trophy wife" because it means the wife is a status symbol, signifying a successful husband. A man with a beautiful wife looks successful in the same way that a man with a beautifully tailored suit or expensive European car looks successful. And that man loves his wife, suit, and car because of the way they make him look.

It can feel strange to be the trophy partner. On one hand, it can seem good to have someone powerful and successful display you like a highly valuable conquest. It means that in the eyes of his social group, *you* have value and status. On the other hand, it feels terrible having someone you love treat you as a status symbol. Add these positive and negative feelings together and you get what psychologists call *ambivalence*. It feels both good and bad and can be confusing.

There's nothing wrong with getting a boost of self-esteem by having an attractive or successful spouse. But if you are in a relationship that's built around being a trophy for your partner, your relationship will become emotionally empty and draining. It requires an enormous amount of work to keep up appearances. In the long run, a relationship based on love, trust, and emotional intimacy is going to do better than one based on status or looks.

While we were visiting with his family, several of us were spending time relaxing outside. Paulo was enjoying the hot tub and I was seated on a lounge chair. As I was speaking to one of his cousins, a woman in a flowery dress walked up behind Paulo, straddled him from behind, pulled his head back, and kissed him on the mouth in front of me!

I wasn't ready for this kind of adulting.

My gut told me something was wrong, but I reasoned, *Maybe this is how adults do it.* I wasn't willing to see the red flag waving right in front of my eyes. Glancing around, wanting to see the reactions of others, I couldn't find anyone who seemed at all alarmed by the absurd behavior.

In our room later that evening, I asked Paulo why he would let that woman kiss him.

"Don't be crazy, Quayle," he chided me. "We've been friends for years. It was harmless. Get over yourself."

Maybe I was crazy.

Back in LA, things returned to normal. At that time, I was along for the ride as long as Paulo was involved. He made me feel special, and I chased that feeling for as long as I could. I didn't realize it then, but Paulo looked at me in a way I'd never experienced before. The look was something more than desire; it was a look of conquest.

> But sometimes we need our eyes to be opened.

When we're in love, when we're vulnerable, we see what we choose to see, we hear what we choose to hear, and we believe what we choose to believe. From firsthand experience, I believe in those moments we're doing the best we can.

But sometimes we need our eyes to be opened.

For further reflection:

- **Notice your patterns of attraction.** Are you naturally attracted to kindness and intimacy, or are you attracted to social status, charisma, and confidence? How have those attraction patterns influenced the course of your relationships?

- **Consider how you get to know a potential romantic partner.** Are you strongly influenced by first impressions, such as the excitement you feel or your gut instinct? Or do you make a more careful analysis by looking at the person's past and seeing how they approach relationships? List some specifics.

- **Pay attention to how long it takes you to "fall" for a partner.** Some people fall in love quickly and move fast. Others are cautious and sometimes miss out on potential relationships. Do you find yourself moving too fast or too slow?

2

IGNORING THE CRACKS

*The Warning Signs We
Choose Not to See*

Quayle, look—your face finally cracked."

When I joined Paulo outside the hangar for coffee, I had just jumped out of the shower. The smell of the jasmine and the cool air was a perfect cocktail for what seemed to be the start of a glorious day, simply being in the moment, feeling grounded on that Saturday morning. I was clean-faced and feeling free in my loose-fitting T-shirt and shorts, ready to take on whatever the day would bring. With a big, self-assured smile, I approached Paulo with open arms in what I thought would be a moment of connection. Instead, it was the opposite. Straight-armed, Paulo stopped my embrace and rejected my hug. He pulled back just enough to take a closer look.

Dismissively, he proclaimed my face had finally cracked.

Like hands pulling a phone away from aging eyes to make out the numbers, he was looking at me as if he might need to get an upgrade.

At the time, I was just twenty-six years old.

What made Paulo's critique particularly disorienting was that most people I met assumed I was much younger than my age. Their response was always, *"You are?"* followed by, *"Oh, I thought you were so much younger!"* Of course, the fact that Paulo's remark about my aging face didn't match with my previous experience didn't lessen the sting of his barb. It was mystifying, hurtful, and burned into my mind with every mirror I faced, every window I passed by on the street, every glance into my rearview mirror, and every room with terrible overhead lighting. Those sharp words caused self-consciousness to fester inside me and take hold. I couldn't shake it off, I couldn't laugh it off, and I couldn't believe he would choose to say something like this to me.

And yet I didn't object.

I didn't retort with my usual "I'll show you" attitude. Instead, I was paralyzed by his words.

I was seventeen years younger than Paulo, and I was already

filled with doubt and insecurities about my age. Those worries had always been that I was too *young* for him. But was I already too old for him?

The clipping of my wings had begun.

WARNING SIGN #1: THE CRITICISM THAT MADE ME CRITICAL OF MYSELF

The criticism didn't stop with Paulo's assessment of my face.

Feeling isolated and alone, with no one to counter his criticisms, I decided I would do what I could do to improve my appearance. I desperately wanted to become someone who would be acceptable to Paulo. So I signed up for a membership at a local gym.

One morning I returned home from a workout, glistening and glowing from within, proud of my new commitment. My cheeks were flushed, and my clothes stained by my sweat and determination. And as I walked in the door, Paulo was making lunch in the kitchen. I was aware of my strength peeking through my tight tank top with a glimpse of maybe a one-pack coming through. I secretly hoped Paulo would notice the results of my hustle and would be proud of my newfound strength in the gym.

Glancing in my direction, Paulo flatly said, "Quayle, looks like you're bulking up."

He could have said anything else. But he said the opposite of what I thought would come out of his mouth. There was no "Atta girl!" Instead, it was the one thing I hoped I'd never hear. His words burned.

Out came the scissors; another wing just got clipped.

If you've been in a toxic relationship, do you remember the first time you were criticized by your partner? Maybe the accusation wasn't that you were "too old" or "too bulky." Maybe the barb that flew toward your heart was that you were too fat, too thin, too controlling, too stupid. And I'm going to venture a guess that the first time you heard it certainly wasn't the *last* time you heard it.

> Paulo's criticism made me critical of myself, and I started to believe I wasn't enough.

The first time Paulo took a shot at my appearance, I had no idea how to respond. Maybe you've felt something similar. You may have also been stunned into silence, unsure how to answer, wading in disbelief or making excuses for what they "really meant to say." Or maybe you knew exactly what you wanted to say, but you also knew, intuitively, it wasn't a safe space to disagree with your partner.

Paulo's criticism made me critical of myself, and I started to believe I wasn't enough.

What's Happening When the Partner Criticizes?

The experience of being criticized by a romantic partner can be painful, especially if an aspect of yourself that you hold dear is being attacked. For example, if you consider yourself intelligent, and your partner says you're stupid; or if you consider yourself attractive, and your partner says you're putting on weight, then the criticism can initially come across as an ego blow. You might feel stunned or confused—even knocked back on your heels a bit. It's so unexpected to hear something negative from someone you think loves you and cares about you that it can feel like a physical blow. The fancy psychological term for this is *ego shock* because it can feel like a brief state of shock or paralysis.

EGO SHOCK: A brief "freezing" of consciousness, psychological numbness, and confusion that can accompany major blows to self-esteem. These blows can include failure, romantic rejection, or humiliation.

A major and unexpected ego blow from someone you love can do psychological damage. You might start to doubt yourself or lose a little faith in your abilities. You might feel a drop in self-esteem or self-worth. It's easy to brush off criticism or defend yourself from someone you don't really care about. We all have strategies, called *defense mechanisms*, to protect our egos from threat.

DEFENSE MECHANISMS: Psychological structures that keep threatening information away from our awareness. Defense mechanisms include *denial*, pretending something didn't happen; *projection*, placing the negative beliefs or emotions onto someone else; or *intellectualization*, where we think rationally about a painful issue but don't allow ourselves to experience the painful emotions.

Logically, we know the people criticizing us don't really know us. Perhaps they are criticizing us from a place of pain, or they're simply trying to put us down to make themselves feel good. But when we are criticized by someone we love, we have to question that person's motives—*Do they really love me?* Or question the relationship—*Is this the loving relationship I thought it was?* Or question our-selves—*Am I really the negative person my partner says I am?* No matter what we conclude—we might agree we are as bad as our partner says, or we might decide our partner does not have our best interest at heart—our relationship is going to be damaged.

WARNING SIGN #2: THE POWER DYNAMICS AT PLAY

"Quayle, your face finally cracked."

"Quayle, looks like you're bulking up."

"Quayle, don't be insecure."

Not long after we met, when Paulo was still introducing me as his "little sister," being called Quayle made me feel special. I liked that he had a nickname for me.

But it also did something else. Calling me his "little sis-ter" and also calling me by my last name—the way a boss might address an underling who was underperforming—signaled the power differential that existed between us. As if it needed any reinforcement. I was never not aware of it. I was twenty-six and he was forty-three. I was female and he was male. I was small and he was big. Any stranger passing us strolling along Venice

Beach, and certainly anyone who'd ever joined us in a conversation, could sense it.

And that's just how Paulo liked it—him being in control.

I didn't realize it at the time, but every time he called me by my last name, it chipped away at my security in the relationship. In the beginning I loved it and saw it as a sign that I was on the inside of his circle. I didn't see how he was grooming me to gradually trust him with this kind of familiarity.

GROOMING: a long-term strategy to gain trust along with physical and emotional intimacy through a series of incremental steps that start out casual and transparent and then become more secretive and close.

Although I didn't understand it at the time, Paulo was continually reinforcing the power dynamic between us. He did it when he'd make comments about how young and inexperienced I was. Ironically, he was also doing it when he signaled that I was visibly aging. He did it when he criticized the appearance of my body. Again and again, he chose to wield his words and actions in ways that made me shrink into silence.

And I did. I never spoke up or spoke out at these verbal power plays. I stayed silent.

Power Dynamics in a Toxic Relationship

On the surface, romantic relationships consist of love, trust, and commitment. But in toxic relationships, underneath this love are destructive power dynamics. Power is all about having control over the partner and their behavior, which can be as simple as selecting which movie to go to or which restaurant to visit or where to go on vacation. These power differentials can be much more toxic when they involve control over finances or sexuality.

In toxic relationships, the toxic partner might try to control you by first gaining your trust and affection, often done via the processes of grooming and love bombing. Grooming is especially common when there is a large power differential between the partners. A boss, professor, priest, or other authority figure who shouldn't be engaging in a romantic relationship in the first place will often start with grooming behaviors that appear innocent. Love bombing involves favorable affection and attention at the beginning of a relationship to overwhelm the partner's natural defenses and any voice in their gut saying this might be toxic.

Once the toxic partner has your full trust and love, they may break down your sense of self-worth or self-esteem by criticizing you or by making you distrust your own sanity, sometimes referred to as *gaslighting*.

GASLIGHTING: A strategy for psychologically manipulating another person into thinking they are going crazy or losing touch with reality.

Once your self-esteem is whittled away and you start to lose trust in your ability to establish reality, you become more vulnerable to being controlled and manipulated. The toxic partner may play games with you by showing romantic interest at times and then removing that interest at other times. For example, they might say, "I love you" one day and then the next day say, "I didn't really mean I love you *that* way." By not being fully committed and playing mind games, the toxic partner maintains power. And as long as you are more interested in maintaining the relationship than your partner is, you'll always sacrifice more and the toxic partner will always maintain power.

A toxic partner may also try to separate you from people who care about you so you don't have outside sources of emotional support or reality testing. If one partner is controlling and isolates the other from social contact and financial support, then eventually, the only place for the partner to get love and affection is from the toxic person. This can create a very negative and hard-to-break dynamic. In a romantic relationship, it can be very difficult to leave.

WARNING SIGN #3: THE FREQUENT FLIRTATIONS

Paulo's backhanded remarks about my appearance weren't the only reason I had to question whether I was good enough for him.

I began to notice Paulo's wandering eyes and the ways he engaged with other women, especially attractive ones or celebrities. Sometimes he'd be particularly friendly with a woman when we were out on a date. Or if he was chatting with a woman at the grocery store, I might sense that there was more happening between them, yet I could never put my finger on it. He never hid his wandering eyes, though. When I'd genuinely and gently inquire about how he had met a particular woman, or what their relationship had been, he'd brush off my careful queries.

Most of my inquiries weren't poorly received by Paulo. In fact, most of them weren't received at all. Rather than hearing my concerns, he would ignore them, brush them off, or accuse me of being insecure and crazy. Not *acting* crazy, just . . . crazy.

Was I simply being insecure as he insisted? Or was my natural intuition, that sense in my gut that something was wrong, doing its job? I didn't know. But I did know that the voice inside my head, whispering that something wasn't right, was getting louder.

One evening, when everything in our relationship was still intoxicating, Paulo and I were seated outside at a little restaurant in Venice. Our server was fair-skinned with auburn hair—a real Jolene type. She was lean and about five feet eight inches tall—everything I wasn't. If I had been out with my girlfriends, I might not have noticed her. But there was something about the looks exchanged between Paulo and the attractive server that made me feel uncomfortable. Their gazes lasted a little too long. If those glances weren't revealing that this pair had a history, they were absolutely hinting that they had a future.

Really? Right in front of me?

I had to go to the bathroom so badly, but I was afraid to leave them alone. Instead, I crossed my legs. I refused to get up and make room for what surely would have been an exchange of phone numbers on a napkin or on the back of a receipt.

I know now that I should have thrown my water at him. I

should have gotten up and said I'd had enough. I should have told him that if he wanted only me, he would have to stop this unacceptable, overt, and disrespectful behavior. But I didn't know *then* what I know *now*.

What I did know then, on some level, was that something wasn't right. And I'm guessing that you've been in similar situations where something inside you—your gut—was telling you that something was off about your partner.

There was a day when I would have been more discerning. The spunky twenty-two-year-old who hadn't yet met Paulo would have called bullshit. But during the course of our relationship, the intuition and gut my parents had instilled in me, through trials and faith, had become hazy somewhere between the I-90 in Montana and the 405 in California. That little voice of intuition had faltered, but it hadn't been extinguished. And it was still trying to let me know something was wrong.

Maybe you've heard that little voice inside, signaling your partner might be involved with someone else. You may have brought it up with your partner and later regretted it. Or you may have sensed it was safer and smarter to silence that voice and suppressed your concern. It's even possible that you chose to keep your concerns from the friends who love you for fear of making your partner look bad.

If you're anything like me, you weren't willing to listen to what that voice was telling you.

Flirtations with Other People (and Trusting Our Gut!)

Many narcissistic partners will look for other potential romantic partners even when they're in a committed relationship. Flirting outside the relationship, or even having romantic affairs, increases their self-esteem, giving them power in their relationship with you because they always have an easy exit. It also keeps them from becoming too committed to your current relationship.

When you're in a relationship with someone who is narcissistic and being flirtatious with others, or even crossing the line into a sexual affair, it's easy to close your eyes in denial. Your partner is unlikely to tell you the truth. Instead, they are more likely to say that you are crazy or insecure or jealous. What your partner is *not* going to say is that they constantly flirt with other people because it makes them feel attractive and important.

If you find yourself in this situation with a potentially unfaithful partner, trust your gut because your gut is far more honest than your partner. However, to find the ultimate source of truth, you either have to become a detective who secretly goes through their partner's life, which is really not healthy for a relationship and doesn't feel good, or you need to start talking to your broader social network and listen to your partner's reputation in that network. If they are running around, there are probably other people who know about it.

You might also look at your partner's dating or relationship history. If your gut is telling you they are cheating and they have a history of doing so, trust your gut at least initially. But if your partner has a history of being faithful and honorable in relationships and in other aspects of their life, it is possible your gut is wrong, and it might be worth a conversation with some friends or even a therapist about where these feelings are coming from.

WARNING SIGN #4: THE BLAME GAME

We were in Punta Mita, Mexico, on a family vacation with friends, and I had gone scuba diving with my friend's little boys. I was in my full wet suit with my mask scrunched up on my forehead, the outline of the mask still imprinted on my face, when I saw *her* from a distance.

Trekking up the beach toward Paulo, pulling the mask off my face, I was certain I looked like a hot mess. Before I spotted Paulo, though, I noticed the raven-haired beauty was standing in the shallow water of the infinity swimming pool, her back to me. Her bright-yellow bikini bottom barely clung to her cheeks as they peeked above the water's surface. The shape of her body made her the perfect specimen of a woman. (Truly, it would take a team of surgeons to get my body to look half as impressive as hers from behind!) As I trudged closer to the pool, I shockingly realized she was face-to-face with Paulo.

Picture this: I'm this disheveled, suction-faced girl, stumbling upon my boyfriend in deep conversation with a younger woman who could have been a supermodel. They were standing too close for having just met. I walked toward them, and my heart raced as I dragged my feet through the sand, listening to the squeaks from my soaking wet suit. I could see that Paulo's charm was on full display. Their flirtatious exchange made me want to run at full speed and wedge myself between them to referee Paulo's game of pretending to be single.

When I finally reached them, he didn't even acknowledge me or introduce me.

While I tried to hold it together on the outside, inside I was pissed. I was embarrassed. I was mortified. There was no way I was going to take off that wet suit so that my body could be compared to hers.

Later that evening in our hotel room, when Eden was off playing with our friends' kids, I asked him about the woman.

"Who was that woman you were talking to in the pool?" I inquired timidly.

Without really answering, he simply said, "Quayle, why are you so crazy? Don't be so insecure."

> "Why are you so crazy? Don't be so insecure."

Well, of course I'm insecure, I argued in my mind, holding myself together because I knew an outburst wouldn't go over well. I thought, *I approached you sporting mask-face and wearing a wet suit while you're talking to the most gorgeous woman in the entire country, and you didn't even acknowledge me or introduce me as your person!*

I felt undone when Paulo would flirt with other women.

For him to call me "crazy" was the easiest, most expedient way to dodge any confrontation or conversation. Blaming me was his default.

Within minutes I'd armored up with a smile to share dinner with our hosts and friends, as if I hadn't just been burned to the ground. As we ate, the Siren—and her fiancé, apparently—were seated just a few tables away. I watched Paulo's gaze find his way to hers—so obvious, so ruthless. And yet I did nothing while my insides were in full combat gear.

From that day forward, whenever he needed to pull out the

"crazy" card, he did it with a derogatory tone that left me wondering if I might actually be crazy. How could the man I loved, whom I had dedicated my life and heart to, whose daughter I'd promised to love like my own, have been so quick to label me crazy and insecure?

He'd said the same of his ex, Eden's mom, which should have been a sign, but I had lost all my footing and any sense of my own boundaries. There was nothing I could say to challenge those two words. Paulo had me in checkmate. My love for him overrode my love for myself, and my self-knowledge. His charm and his version of the truth convinced me I was the problem. He claimed I needed to work on myself. I started to believe him, and the flame that once burned brightly in my soul became a flicker.

> His charm and his version of the truth convinced me I was the problem.

It hadn't been easy for me to initiate conversations I knew had the potential to set Paulo off. But when I did gather my courage to bring up a difficult topic, the result was fairly predictable. My concerns were dismissed. They were unheard. The substance of them was never discussed. Instead, I was labeled and blamed. Why? Because if I was insecure, then Paulo didn't have to take responsibility for his behavior. If I was crazy, then he could dismiss any legitimate concerns I had.

WARNING SIGN #5: THE LIMITED INPUT
FROM THOSE WHO KNEW HIM

Today, I would see the signs.

I've learned that one of the ways we can gather insightful information about a partner is by spending time with them in the presence of the people who know them and care about them. And while I loved spending time with Eden, we both had similar experiences of Paulo: we knew only what he wanted us to know about him. And the life that Paulo and I shared didn't leave room for me to gather the kind of information that would add to my understanding of who he was. I didn't know his family. The relationships I had with his friends were surface-level and guarded. At the end of the day, they were his friends; therefore, they'd protect him and his secrets at any cost.

I only had Paulo.

Even the whole business about him living in an airplane hangar—living the single life as if he had everything figured out—may have been a way for Paulo to escape from the real world and do whatever he wanted, far from the eyes of others. This was just one of the ways he lived recklessly.

In the absence of relationships with people who knew Paulo well, I saw what he wanted me to see.

Of course, hindsight is twenty-twenty, but in retrospect, I now know how I could have acted differently. I can see how I

Of course, hindsight is twenty-twenty, but in retrospect, I now know how I could have acted differently.

could have discovered who Paulo was long before I *actually* discovered who Paulo was.

I could've pursued opportunities to know people in his family.

I could've taken the opportunity to build a relationship with Eden's mother, inviting her to speak honestly.

I could've built relationships with the friends who came around. And even if they didn't throw him under the bus, I could have learned *something* from them.

That's a lot of *could'ves*, I know. But the blessing is that what I didn't get right back then, I can now share with you so you can spend less time questioning yourself.

When the person with whom we're in a toxic relationship is the one source of information we have about them, that person controls the narrative. We know only what they tell us. We know only the parts of them they allow us to see. And they can be savvy about what they share.

Recognizing a Narcissist

Narcissistic partners don't wear T-shirts advertising this trait. In fact, narcissism is a combination of overly positive self-views, energy, and assertiveness—all positive qualities in a partner, and initially quite attractive—mixed with a strong sense of entitlement, superiority, and self-importance.

NARCISSISM: a personality trait describing an inflated sense of oneself along with a relative lack of compassion or empathy for other people. Narcissists can manipulate and exploit others and have a powerful craving for attention and admiration.

People who are narcissistic will have a pattern of relationships that start out positively and end up with infidelity or deception. They will also have troubled family relationships and troubled business relationships. When you look at their history, you will see patterns of drama.

The narcissist isn't going to tell you about any of this, and if you do learn about a negative past, the narcissist will likely say it's because of somebody else's fault. And they will explain this dramatic story in a convincing way. It's important to remember that you cannot take a narcissist's word for reality or the truth. In order to understand them, you need to speak with family members, old business partners, and especially old relationship partners, if possible. There may be a lot of mystery surrounding this person.

Given how difficult it is to understand what you're getting into with a narcissist, especially one who's charming and charismatic, I'd strongly suggest *slowing down*. You don't need to get married in six months. If this relationship is meant to be, it can handle a little thought and time at the beginning to really get to know each other. Do your due diligence before committing. Look at this person rationally and pragmatically to see if their words match their actions. Check references.

As my relationship with Paulo continued, the vibrant, outspoken girl I'd once been became smaller. I lost myself. I shrank. My confident "I'll show you" attitude was replaced with self-doubt.

And I even began to believe, *Maybe I'm the problem.*

For further reflection:

- **Build your trust network.** Think about people in your life whom you trust to offer you smart, honest, and loving feedback about your relationships, like a parent, sibling, best friend, or therapist. What could you do to strengthen or grow that network?

- **Recognize good and bad relationships.** It's difficult to recognize a bad relationship as it begins. Think about your friends who have healthy romantic relationships and those who gravitate toward more unhealthy, toxic ones. What do you think resulted in those different relationship outcomes? What warning signs were there from the beginning? Now reflect on your relationship history. What warning signs did you see? What red flags did you miss?

- **Trust yourself.** We all have skills, insights, and wisdom that people seek from us. Think about some of these strengths that you have and those areas where you have the most confidence. What decisions are you good at making? What wisdom or skills do you have that people seek from you?

3

GASLIGHTING 101

*The Ways We're Convinced
to Rewrite the Story*

t was New Year's Eve and I was eager to share it with
the man to whom I'd given my heart.

The evening began with a lavish dinner at the hangar
with another couple. I use the word *couple* loosely because the
woman who was sharing festive drinks with Paulo's friend Greg
was neither Greg's wife nor the mother of his children. *Do Greg
and his wife have an open relationship? Does she know where he
is? Does she have someone else too?*

I had no way of knowing. I'd learned that it was dangerous to ask questions, so I stayed silent. Quelling my own discomfort so that others would be comfortable, I tried to convince myself that Greg's business was none of mine. After all, I was deep in my own relationship where my footing was slipping. Most days I felt like I was walking on a high wire in high heels—backward, blindfolded. With every step I took, I faltered a little more.

Throughout the evening, I was curious about Greg's marriage, but more than I wanted answers, I wanted to keep the peace.

Looking back, I can see some of the ways I was being gaslighted.

WAY #1: WE'RE CONVINCED TO IGNORE OUR GUT

Still in my twenties, I was relatively new to adulthood. I hadn't had great, healthy relationships with men, so I didn't know what was normal behavior and what was me being uptight or not understanding. Therefore, I stifled the little voice inside me that knew something wasn't right. I convinced myself I was the one with the problem. Tell a girl she's insecure and crazy enough times, and she'll probably start to believe you.

Have you heard that little voice inside you before? The one that whispers something isn't right? That voice, that knowing in our gut, is for our good. And yet when we sense that heeding this voice might cause trouble for us, we ignore it. We silence it. We do what we must to not make waves.

After our starter drinks at the hangar, the four of us piled into Paulo's black four-door Cadillac truck: men in the front, women in the back. We were heading to Hotel Angeleno for a New Year's Eve bash at the Penthouse Bar. This refurbished Holiday Inn had become a place where the who's who of yesteryear came for overpriced bottle service and chilled drinks in a special roped-off VIP section that garnered lots of attention. It was the kind of place where people go to be seen; everyone was looking around to see who might be looking at them—a classic LA kind of night. This was an older crowd, filled with jaded perennial guest stars, bitter from seeing their roles going to people less qualified.

I'd always had a rocky relationship with vodka, using it to drown my latest mistake or soothe a recent heartbreak. But because it was the beginning of a new year, I decided that maybe vodka and I would reconcile. After all, it was the only choice in our bottle service, and my cup runneth over. I hadn't eaten much during the day in an effort to fit into the clingy dress hugging my humble curves and

> Tell a girl she's insecure and crazy enough times, and she'll probably start to believe you.

be what I thought Paulo wanted. Not a good idea in a place where glasses were never empty, and water was nowhere to be found.

Around that time Paulo had been distracted, and he'd been treating me more unkindly than usual. But I desperately wanted to believe in the fairy-tale notion that the countdown to midnight and the magical turn-of-the-year kiss would break the evil spell we'd been under. I wanted to believe he'd love me again like he first did. As we danced and laughed, it *did* feel like we were turning a new page. This, I wanted to believe, would be when we got back to *us*. We were set up and on track for an amazing night. Love and heat filled the lounge as everyone enthusiastically awaited the chance to enter a new year in a cloud of spirited smoke . . . and mirrors.

Then, in what felt like a punch to my gut, I noticed Paulo making his way across the crowded room. He was at it again. Chatting up another woman and looking at her in the way he'd once looked at me. His prowess was on full display. The object of Paulo's attention had been a famous young actress from the eighties, still beautiful and thin. Everyone was watching her, but my eyes were on him. Reaching for another drink, my heart dissolved into another glass of vodka on ice with a splash of soda and lime.

When he finally rejoined our group, I was emboldened by liquid courage.

"What are you doing?" I asked with an edge to my voice. "Why do you need to talk to her? You're here with me."

And then he acted out his script yet again, attacking me with verbal guns blazing and doubling down on shaming me. Once again, I was crazy and insecure.

"Quayle," he hissed, "you're making up stories again."

The Story Behind Gaslighting

There was a popular psychological thriller movie in the 1940s called *Gaslight*. It tells the story of a woman who falls into a whirlwind romance and marriage to a husband who isn't as honorable as he seems. To control and manipulate his wife, the husband engages in a campaign that makes her believe she is losing her mind. For example, he makes strange noises in the house and adjusts the gaslights up and down. When she questions him about the changes in the gaslights, he denies anything is happening and suggests that she might be losing her mind.

This form of manipulation is now popularly described as *gaslighting*. This isn't to be confused with two people seeing a situation differently, but rather it involves *intentionally* denying reality to make someone question their own sanity, doubt themselves, create confusion, and cause them to lose confidence in their decision-making ability. Gaslighting is a subtle yet powerful way to psychologically control someone or to get away with something because it weakens the victim's sense of what is real and what isn't. As a result, gaslighting makes people more susceptible to abuse and manipulation.

When the victims of gaslighting start to lose their firm grasp on reality, they can become more dependent on the gaslighter, making them even more vulnerable to manipulation. Therefore, it's important to recognize the signs of gaslighting: blatant lying, denying, instilling confusion, questioning your sanity, projecting (accusing you of their wrongdoing), discrediting your memory of events, and trivializing. Trust your gut and your senses. If things feel off or look off, trust that they might *be* off—even if your partner says you are being silly, childish, or paranoid. It's also important to seek some form of outside support if you think you might be a victim of gaslighting. Having a few close friends, family members, or advisors you can trust to tell you the truth will help you stay grounded in reality.

WAY #2: WE'RE CONVINCED
WE'RE OVERREACTING

That night I had been bolder than usual with my queries. When I was sober, I was more cautious about questioning or challenging Paulo. Knowing that I'd often be accused of overreacting, I tried to keep my reactions, my wonderings, my questions, and my concerns small. To appease Paulo, I made *myself* small—again.

What I'd learned was that it was safer to ignore my instincts—to silence my inner voice, to ignore my gut.

Maybe you learned the same thing. When we are being careful not to overreact, we play it small. Not only do we modulate ourselves from appearing to overreact, but we also keep ourselves from expressing the normal kinds of reactions that situations might warrant. A part of us knows our concerns are valid, but we go along to get along.

Your Gut: The Second Brain

Believe it or not, our gut can work like a second brain. It can pick up on social and environmental threats and opportunities, and respond with physical sensations that eventually become emotions. For example, we might feel queasy or experience butterflies in our stomach when we're in a dangerous or uncomfortable situation. Disgust, in particular, has a strong connection with our gut; something might make us want to vomit, which is an indication we should stay away from it. This "little brain" in our gut is called the *enteric nervous system* (ENS).

Sometimes the story we tell ourselves is not the whole story, and we may miss out on some real threats. That's when our gut starts giving us different messages. Although our gut communicates with feelings, it's often wise to listen to that little brain's voice and see if it's providing us with accurate information. The gut doesn't know everything and isn't always correct, but it always makes sense to stop and listen seriously to what it is saying.

WAY #3: THE BLAME SHIFTS

Paulo's New Year's Eve flirtation with the beautiful actress wasn't anything new. A slideshow of faces cascaded through my mind in that moment—including the brunette waitress in Venice, the Mexico beach beauty, and countless others. In each case, when I was accused of overreacting, the intuition that had been ignited in me, for the briefest of moments, was eventually doused. In the storm of Paulo's denials, shaming, and gaslighting, I'd eventually concede. I was wrong. I was too sensitive. He was right.

Whenever I'd gather my courage to ask about one of the countless other women to whom he showed attention, he'd dismiss me with, "Here you go again, Quayle . . ."

It wasn't just that I was the person *with* the problem. He always seemed to frame it to communicate to me that I *was* the problem.

When someone denies what seems obvious, it's a little confusing, isn't it? And that confusion is underscored when they're loud in their defense, when they're insistent, when they're belligerent, and when they point the finger at us—saying we're the problem—they often refuse to take any responsibility for their own behavior.

Often, those outside the situation can see it better than we can. They notice that it looks like a pig and smells like a pig. Meanwhile, we're wondering, *Am I the pig?* When Paulo called me "insecure" and "crazy," he wasn't just saying that he disagreed with me—he was dismissing me, because if I were crazy, then anything I said was irrelevant.

The Dreaded Trigger Words

When you are being gaslighted by someone, their goal is to make you feel insecure about yourself and question your own sense of reality. In the process, you might hear certain terms or phrases such as, "You're acting *crazy!*" or "Stop being so *insecure.*" or "This is nonsense. You're acting *silly.*" Your partner might make you feel childish, inexperienced, or immature, as if you don't understand relationships. You might even be called "paranoid" or be told that you are "losing it." Often, the abusive and toxic partner assumes the role of a scolding parent to make you feel ashamed, insecure, or stupid.

"Quayle," Paulo snapped as the New Year's Eve festivities carried on, "you're going to ruin everything!"

Then, pulling something out of his pocket, Paulo instructed, "Take these."

Reaching for my hand, he sprinkled some small objects into my palm.

Looking down, I saw a few pills of different colors and something that looked like a mashed-up mushroom. Paulo closed my hand and gave me a look that said, *Don't ruin this.*

I understood the assignment.

I went to the bathroom, hand clenched and heart broken. In the stall, I locked the door and opened my hand. His words of blame echoed in my mind louder than all the noise of high heels on tile and slurred conversations in the bathroom that night. It was as if these little pills of persuasion in the palm of my clammy hand spelled "ruin," yet I took them all at once with only my determination to wash them down.

Although I had never done drugs before, I convinced myself that I had nothing to lose. This, I believed, would make Paulo happy with me. *Just do what he says.* In my head I kept replaying Paulo's words, *Quayle, you're going to ruin everything!* So I took that handful of so-called fun, not knowing what he gave me. I swallowed them all dry, then came out of the stall, looked at my twenty-eight-year-old face, and told myself to pull it together. As soon as the other girls who were fixing their lipstick had left me alone with my own reflection, I pointed at myself in the mirror and said, "Don't you ruin this, Quayle."

Thirty minutes later, after rejoining the group, I was finding it difficult to stand. I sat down on the soft velvet seating in our roped-off area amid a clutter of empty bottles. My body began to sway, and my eyes began losing focus.

Let's just say that Paulo and I never made it to the happy new year I'd imagined we'd ring in.

Paulo and our friends realized they needed to get me out of there, or it was going to be a situation of police proportion. If they didn't leave promptly, others might notice my condition and start to ask questions. So they swept me toward the exit and sat me down on a cold metal bench outside the hotel as we waited for the valet to pull up.

When the valet arrived with Paulo's truck, Greg, who was the *least* intoxicated among us, drove us back to the hangar. As we sped down the 405, I yelled that Paulo was trying to kill me, begging Greg and his female friend to protect me from him. Then I rolled down the window and attempted to jump out of the vehicle. They pulled me in and, thankfully, my delicate heart never felt the highway.

Back at Paulo's hangar, he carried me upstairs and sat me in a cold shower with my clothes still clinging to my limp body, which was trying to rid itself of the poison it had been given.

My most vivid memory of that night was begging, "Please don't let him kill me. He's trying to kill me!"

WAY #4: WE'RE SABOTAGED

When I think back to the younger me in the bathroom stall that night, it breaks my heart. She was trying so hard to do all the right things, but nothing was ever good enough.

I can't say what Paulo intended when he gave me those pills. There is no way to know for sure. But I *can* say for certain that it was not for my good. As I reflect back, I would like to think he was just looking to have a numbingly good time. But his carelessness for my safety and my recklessness in taking unknown substances could have taken my life.

Toxic partners, if they have a heart, have one only for themselves. My partner gave me pills that put my life at risk. Another partner takes his wife's car from the parking lot while she's at work. And another cleans out his girlfriend's bank account. Yet another ostracizes his partner's friends. These toxic and abusive partners sabotage our well-being.

On the morning of January 1, my body hurt all over as if I had been punched from the inside out. My ribs and abs ached from all the vomiting and heaving. My hair was a mess from being hosed down and was clumped against my head. My eye makeup was still visible under my eyes, and my cheeks were stained with a mix of tears and mascara.

Paulo wouldn't look at me, much less apologize for poisoning me. It was all anger. He didn't speak to me for almost a week. I was the one who ended up apologizing. I was in ruins.

Once again, he was wrong, but I was the one who was punished.

The Subtle Sabotage

In order to control or manipulate in a relationship, someone who is sociopathic, psychopathic, or narcissistic may try to break you down mentally or emotionally until you become insecure, isolated, and easy to control. This formula can be seen in cults where people join for positive reasons but are eventually separated or cut off from the world, along with their family and friends, receiving outside messages only in a controlled environment from the cult leader.

Similarly, narcissistic, sociopathic, psychopathic, and abusive individuals in romantic relationships use the same process of indirectly sabotaging their partner's self-esteem, self-confidence, or self-worth to gain power. In addition to gaslighting, this can also be achieved through making the partner feel stupid by calling out their mistakes and not offering credit for their successes.

For someone being sabotaged, it's crucial that this person is unaware of what's happening and ideally cut off from outside forms of support. The saboteur doesn't want the partner's best friend or mother to tell them that they're being manipulated, so the saboteur will keep the partner away from others and make them believe they are the only person who knows what's best for them.

If you find yourself in a relationship with someone who appears confident and self-assured, yet you feel your own sense of confidence and self-esteem slipping away—and if you find yourself cut off from all your old sources of social support and affection—you might be a victim of sabotage in a relationship. Healthy relationships prioritize honesty, trust, and genuine concern for each partner's well-being.

WAY #5: WE'RE CONVINCED TO MAKE EXCUSES

When Paulo's behaviors started changing, I'd make excuses for him.

Not long after New Year's, my dad called to check and see how I was doing. Largely, I hid my life with Paulo from my family. If I didn't visit home, then they couldn't see what I didn't want them to see. But they still knew, somehow.

"What is he doing with you?" my dad asked. "He should be jumping at the opportunity to marry you and start a family with you."

"Be patient, Dad," I'd beg. "He's definitely going to ask me to marry him. He just needs more time."

I made up excuses for Paulo with my family. I made excuses for his ugly behavior with my friends. Whenever anyone would question Paulo, I'd insist that he was in the right. If anyone was in the wrong, I'd assure them it was me.

In toxic relationships, rather than protecting ourselves, we protect our partners. We might do it publicly, offering onlookers a plausible excuse for why they are behaving badly. Or we might do it in private, assuring a well-meaning friend that they were overworked, or drank too much, or was upset about something else. We make excuses to preserve the relationship, but it often comes at a cost.

Making Excuses for Bad Behavior

We often tell ourselves an idealized story about our romantic relationships: it's positive and growing in a healthy direction; and our partner is a loving, beautiful person. But sometimes that story isn't correct; our partner is *not* loving and does *not* have our best interest at heart, and the relationship is *not* healthy.

It's not easy to change a story once we have it in place. So when we see behaviors that don't fit with our beautiful story, we make excuses. For example, if our partner puts us down, we might remain silent and tell ourselves they are just trying to make us a better person with their feedback. To keep the story of the healthy relationship alive, we add another story that we deserve abuse.

There is a psychological term for this: cognitive dissonance.

COGNITIVE DISSONANCE: the discomfort we experience when our beliefs don't line up with the reality we experience.

There are a few different ways we can get rid of this uncomfortable cognitive dissonance in our relationships. We can tell ourselves a different story. We can admit the relationship partner isn't a good person, and our beautiful relationship really isn't so. This kind of honesty is hard because it means giving up our idealized story. So instead of being honest with ourselves, the more natural way to resolve cognitive dissonance initially is to make excuses for the behaviors that don't fit into our fantasy. When our partner is abusive, we instead blame ourselves or make some other excuse for their bad behavior.

If you find yourself in a relationship where you're constantly making excuses for your partner, and the story you're telling yourself about the relationship doesn't seem to match up with the reality, then you might be in a state of cognitive dissonance. Just like with gaslighting, it is important to seek advice and insight from someone you trust outside the relationship. Doing so will prevent you from making excuses for your partner's behavior and covering up the toxic relationship.

For further reflection:

- **Trust your gut.** Think about your gut as a little brain that can intuitively detect subtle and overt behaviors. What does your gut tell you about your relationship? Does your relationship sit well for you or does it make you a little queasy when you think about it?

- **Understand who you are.** One of the best defenses against being sabotaged or manipulated in a relationship is to have a very solid understanding of who you are as a person. What are your greatest strengths? What do you value? What do others value about you?

- **Recognize and avoid gaslighting.** It can be difficult to see gaslighting, narcissism, or abuse in our own life, but it is often obvious when we look at the relationships of our friends, colleagues, family members, or even some of the relationships we see in the media. Reflect on some gaslighting examples you've witnessed in other relationships. Why did the victim allow the abuse to happen? How might the individual have gotten out of that destructive situation?

4

SECRETS REVEALED
AND LIES OUT
IN THE OPEN

The Questions We Can't Avoid

There's been an accident. You better come quickly."
It was a friend calling from the hangar.

I'd just started cooking dinner for Paulo and Eden before showering off after my run and getting ready for my show with my band. Eden was in our bedroom watching TV with the dogs. The oil sizzled in the pan as I sautéed Paulo's favorite veggies for fajitas. He would be home at any moment, and I wanted the smell in our tiny shotgun kitchen to fill him with the fragrance of love and devotion.

Tossing down my spatula, I ran to twelve-year-old Eden.

"We have to go. Your dad's been in an accident."

I've always been able to drive fast, but that night my car had wings. I called my dad on our way down the Pacific Coast Highway in that little Volkswagen Jetta with our nerves hanging on by a thread and our hearts beating wildly. Not knowing what we were about to encounter, I darted in and out of lanes as we made our way to the Santa Monica Airport. *Did I put the car in park? Did I leave the keys in the ignition?* We ran separately, together. We were running, then we were screaming, then we were being held back by policemen. They wouldn't let us get any closer.

Paulo was dead. And I had questions.

QUESTION #1: IS EVERYONE IN ON A JOKE AND THE PUNCHLINE IS ME?

The morning of the public memorial service, I had been going on four straight days without sleep. After dousing my brain with caffeine, I put on my black dress. I got Paulo's dog, Flaca, in his truck and left our house to pick up Eden in Marina del Rey. My parents would meet us at the Santa Monica Airport, as would Eden's mom, stepdad, and little brother.

As we pulled into the airport parking lot, the trauma of

the last time Eden and I had arrived there together hit us. I squeezed her hand. Before I left our house, I'd taken half of a Xanax to help me not fall apart so I could be there for her like I had been the night of the plane crash. I didn't want to lose it in front of her or anyone else, so I dulled my pain just enough.

As we slowly walked through the slatted metal gate, the smell of roses stung my nose. The fragrance was so sweet it sickened me. Red rose petals had been scattered on the smooth concrete floor around each plane to honor his life lost on that unbelievably tragic day. A small, gray-carpeted stage had been set up facing the runway with a simple microphone and speaker. This is where we would address the crowd. Inside the hangar we had put together a slideshow of our life together: videos and photographs of memories projected on the wall, from family vacations to us just being us. The slideshow had included my favorite photo of the three of us swimming with dolphins, one of Paulo sporting a big smile behind his aviators in the cockpit of the plane, a video of us and the dogs on our property overlooking the Valley from the Airstream, the photo of Paulo and me in our matching champagne-colored suit and dress from a night celebrating at a club together. It was *us* in an eight-minute slideshow on repeat.

Underneath my black dress, my body was wasting away. A sudden inability to eat had come with my grief. I was

> I was a woman in mourning but not a widow.

struggling with my role. I was a woman in mourning but not a widow. *What am I?* I don't think there was a defining title for what I was other than heartbroken, grieving, and emotionally destroyed.

As droves of people began arriving, I noticed Eden was clenching her eulogy in her hands. I stayed close to her and she to me. I held on to my paper too, as if this tribute might be ripped from my grasp.

"Who are all these people?" we said to one another.

Neither of us recognized most of the hundreds who'd gathered to remember Paulo's life.

Leaning toward my ear, Eden admitted, "I don't think I wanna get up and speak."

I felt the same.

"You know what?" I offered. "I don't want to either. Let's save our words for the smaller family service."

We agreed to save our speeches until the private family funeral, set to take place in two days at the church at Eden's school.

As we wandered through the throng of people, I passed a trio of women I'd never seen before.

One of them lowered her voice but still spoke a bit too loudly, saying, "If he hadn't died, I would have totally had a chance with him. She's not that pretty."

My edges were dulled by the small dose of Xanax, but my eyes and ears registered disbelief. This wasn't the first time women talked about me behind my back, or even in front of me. But this was my boyfriend's memorial service! *Who are all these women anyway?*

I was his person and Eden was his daughter, but we were swimming in a sea of strangers.

Remember the People on Your Side

In the midst of chaos, real love is often sitting right beside you—patient, quiet, and steadfast—among your true friends and family. These are the people who will stand by you through the good times and bad. When you enter into an exciting but potentially toxic romantic relationship, your ability to make smart decisions for yourself and your future becomes compromised. Your friends and family can often see what's going on. They know it's a bad relationship, or at least has a lot of downsides. They can see through the lies of a slippery romantic partner much more easily than you can. They are not sucked into romance or overwhelmed with emotions; therefore, they can see much more clearly.

Unfortunately, when you are in the thrall of a romantic relationship, it's difficult to hear a message from friends or family when they tell you it isn't the right relationship. The conversation rarely goes well. You might go to great lengths to defend your relationship or turn your back on friends and family for love, even if that romance turns out to be toxic.

It's important not to destroy old friendships and family relationships. If your romantic relationship ultimately falls apart, your true friends and family are going to be there to help you pick up the pieces. Some might say "I told you so" and get frustrated—it can be tough to watch a friend stay in a bad relationship when it's so clear from the outside—but oftentimes you will find love and acceptance, along with relief that you are out of a bad situation. These are the people who deserve your appreciation and credit. When you find those people, treasure them.

QUESTION #2: WHO WAS THIS PERSON I WAS WITH?

Shortly after sunset, I was back at the house in the small courtyard, sitting on the rounded concrete fixture, the ashtray overflowing with half-smoked cigarettes. My friend Michelle stood by with her watchful eye. My stepmom, Loretta, wanted me to stop smoking but knew now was not the time to attempt this conversation; smoking helped numb my pain.

The back door opened without warning. It was one of my closest friends, looking angrier than I had ever seen her. As I lit what must have been my hundredth cigarette that day, she came out to the courtyard and said, "You have to move on."

"What are you talking about?" I whimpered in my shell of a voice. "I'm still working with the coroner on his dental records. I can't move on."

"A girl came up to me at the funeral and introduced herself as Paulo's girlfriend. She said they were supposed to meet next weekend during the Super Bowl party but that 'God had other plans.'"

I didn't inhale. I didn't exhale. I was covered in smoke, and my grieving heart started to unravel into the darkest feeling of betrayal I had ever known. In an instant, anger lodged in my heart while grief quickly found its compartment and slammed the door. There was no room for sadness anymore. I had been betrayed. I was a fool. And how long had everyone else known? In that moment, I finally came to terms with my gut question: *Who can I trust?*

Piecing Together the Person You Thought You Knew

We all go through life acting a bit like psychologists—building models, profiles, or character studies of the people closest to us. This personality model-building starts when we first learn about trusting other people and develops into more complex models.

Sometimes our models are wrong—even wildly so. Misjudgment or mischaracterization is particularly common in relationships with narcissists. The more toxic qualities are often hidden, and we start off with a very positive model. When the betrayal happens—when you find out that your "perfect and loving" partner has been cheating on you—that model collapses. That person was not at all who you thought they were.

Realizing you were so wrong about your partner can be devastating in many ways. You were in a loving relationship with a dishonest person, and you didn't see it. All those beautiful memories weren't as beautiful as you once thought. A lot of what you thought was so special and wonderful was really a lie. This is a powerful blow to anyone's sense of reality. On top of the confusion and betrayal, there can be a sense of shame or embarrassment. *Why didn't I see this quality or the false side of my partner? How could everyone else see it and I couldn't?*

What I often tell people is that it is *very* hard to detect narcissism, psychopathy, and other toxic traits when you fall in love with somebody, especially if the narcissistic partner is manipulating you by love bombing or gaslighting, or if the person has more wealth or power than you and has more control over the relationship.

When betrayal happens, the best strategy is often to accept the truth, even if it is painful. This can take some processing, and it's important to maintain self-compassion along the way. Be kind to yourself and realize that many people end up in this situation and come through it. Don't feel like the abuse you endured was your fault. It wasn't. Think of it as something to learn from and avoid in the future.

QUESTION #3: WHAT DOES IT SAY ABOUT
ME THAT I WAS WITH THIS PERSON?

The house had its own presence, and up until Sunday evening it had been one of loving sadness. But as I learned the truth, the house did too, and soon there was an eerie darkness that thickened the rooms. It seemed like every hair on my body was standing at attention from the hostile energy. There was an ever-present feeling that someone was watching me. But I was angry, and my anger pushed me through the unease. I went into Paulo's office to get his computer from his briefcase. I brought it into the dining room where Michelle and my step-mom were, and I plugged the cord into the socket to the left of the double-sided fireplace. The sound of it powering on rang in my ears.

The photos . . . I started there and saw things I can never unsee. Burned into my memories are all the women, photos taken by him, of them: brunettes, blondes. There was no parti-cular type; the common denominator was they were in his bed, in his pictures, wearing nothing but a look of yearning for him to put the camera down.

I wanted to throw up, but I also wanted to get to the bottom of what I had just seen.

I attached my hard drive cable to his computer and went to the screen to click "download." But before I ever got into his emails, I slammed the computer shut and pushed myself back in the chair to get as far away as possible from it.

Our home had been my refuge, but now it felt unsafe.

How had I fallen for this ruse? I was flooded by feelings of guilt and shame.

Maybe you've felt something similar. When we feel guilt, we feel like what's happened is our fault. And when we feel shame, we feel like there's something wrong with *us*. While I didn't know it at the time, nothing could be further from the truth.

Shame and Guilt

Responsible, conscientious people will often take responsibility for their relationship when it falls apart. But when you're in a relationship with a narcissist, they will make sure that you take the blame. The psychological term for this is called the *self-serving bias* or taking credit for success and blaming the other for failure. This is also part of gaslighting. For example, the narcissist will say something like, "I'm doing a great job in this relationship. The reason I'm cheating on you is because you're not attractive enough and you're not fun enough." The narcissist will take your natural desire or inclination for responsibility and use that as a tool to manipulate you. The next thing you know, you are blaming yourself for your partner's toxic behavior.

Psychologically speaking, there's an important difference between guilt and shame. Guilt is that negative feeling we get when we break a social rule. We might feel guilty if we are caught speeding or if we stay out too late partying and can't go to work in the morning. Guilt can be resolved by apology and remedial action: say you're sorry, pay the fine, and go on with life.

Shame, however, is when you think you are fundamentally flawed or broken, someone who can't help but do things wrong. Shame can be damaging because there's no easy way to get rid of it. But here's the good news: you are not a fundamentally bad person. So if you were feeling shame beyond that which is normal, it might be best tackled with a psychotherapist or counselor. When we get in an ashamed mindset, it's hard to see our value, and sometimes having an outsider bring clarity makes it easier.

QUESTION #4: IT WASN'T JUST ME
HE WAS LYING TO, WAS IT?

By the time I fell into bed Sunday night, I had the faces of countless women in my mind who'd likely been with Paulo while we were dating. As I lay awake, a fury welled up inside me as I thought about the risk to which he'd exposed me. I wasn't taking any chances.

First thing on Monday morning, Loretta accompanied me to an emergency visit to the gynecologist.

Paulo had left with me with so much pain, but what else might he have left me with? He had been with numerous women, and for how long I didn't know. *Will this be the end of me?* I wondered. *What if I'm pregnant? What if I won't be able to have kids? What if he left me with a lifelong reminder in the form of a disease?*

Seated by my stepmom, waiting for my name to be called in the waiting room of the doctor's office, I was screaming inside. Hiding behind my sunglasses, feeling like damaged goods, I felt so full of shame.

"Everything looks okay," the doctor confirmed. "We'll call you within the week if any of your tests come back positive." When the phone rang from my doctor's office several days later stating that I was in the clear, a feeling of gratitude washed over me.

Despite the fact that I was well physically, the evidence of these women had convinced me that everything I had been suspecting was true. I wasn't insecure. I wasn't crazy. He was a narcissist, a sociopath, a psychopath, a *liar*.

My stepmom and I went to Venice Beach for a coffee, and I hid in agony and anger behind my sunglasses. I still didn't have the final records from the coroner confirming that Paulo had been in the single-engine plane that crashed shortly after take-off on the west end of the runway and then caught on fire. His Blackberry had been retrieved from the crash, but it was his dental records that would give final confirmation that it was, in fact, Paulo who had died.

There were some theories that the plane had been tampered with—or that maybe Paulo had faked his own death. After all, there had been another man in the plane as well. But it was the dental records that provided the final confirmation, which allowed me to begin my process of letting go.

The private funeral was set for the following Tuesday. Michelle was my caretaker and ran interference for me in the days leading up to it. I wasn't taking anyone's calls; Loretta's loving silence was the only comfort I could stand. I answered the phone only for Mary, Eden's mom. She called as I sipped my bitter coffee while holding back tears to ask if she could take Paulo's computer so Eden could get photos of her dad.

"You can have whatever you want," I said flatly.

She must have recognized the deadness in my tone.

"You found out . . ." Mary began.

But I spoke at the same moment. "You knew?"

It was as much an accusation as it was an observation.

"Stef," she pled, "I wanted to tell you, but you wouldn't have believed me because he'd convinced you that I was this crazy ex. He convinced you like he had convinced so many others."

As much as I wanted her to be wrong, I knew she wasn't. But I still wish I'd been given the opportunity to hear about Paulo's true nature and then decide for myself.

She went on to say that she figured telling me he was cheating would have led me to lean in even closer to him. We'll never know what I would have done; I wasn't given that option. Maybe it's because I was Eden's caretaker when she wasn't with her mom, and Mary knew Eden was safe with me.

Untangling a Web of Lies

Personality psychologists have a saying: "The best predictor of future behavior is past behavior." This is another way of saying that people are consistent in their behavior across time and situation. If you cheated on people in the past, you're likely to cheat in the future.

If you're lying about one or two things, you're probably lying about more.

Here is another way to think about it: If you catch your partner lying, do you think you caught them in the only lie they told? What are the odds that you were able to detect their single lie? It's difficult to know when people are lying, and even trained detectives can't do it well; that's why the detectives will have suspects repeat their story over and over, to try to find inconsistencies. And if you are with somebody who makes a habit out of lying, they are probably skilled at deception. Plus, you love and trust the person, which makes you easier to deceive. In new, exciting relationships it's going to be hard to detect lies, and if you do detect one, chances are there are even more that you didn't.

Let's be clear: This doesn't mean people can't change. Part of becoming an adult and maturing is taking responsibility for yourself and being more honest and forthright. That being said, people tend to be consistent in their behavior, so if somebody lies to you once about something important, it's reasonable to suspect they will do it again. In fact, if you've noticed people lie to others, chances are they will be willing to lie to you as well. That's why many people don't do business with people who cheat on their spouses. Can someone be trusted in a business relationship if they can't be trusted in a marriage?

For further reflection:

- **Choose to see well.** Falling in love and seeing the best in your partner is healthy and positive, but it also has risks. In your past relationships, have there been times when rose-colored glasses—or seeing the best in another—were helpful? Were there other times when you were blind to a partner's toxic behaviors?

- **Learn from healthy relationships.** In the healthy relationships around you, notice how each partner in the relationship relates to the other. Do they idealize one another? Or do they really know one another deeply like close friends or family? Or is it a combination?

- **Learn from toxic relationships.** How do individuals in unhealthy relationships relate to each other? If one of your friends remains in a toxic relationship, what do you think your friend sees in their partner that other people don't? Are they blinded to negative things their partner does? How do they exaggerate the positive aspects of their partner to cover up the negative?

5

HIS TRUTH, MY TRUTH, THE TRUTH

The Ways We Start to Make Sense of the Chaos

For years, I'd imagined Eden and I walking down the aisle of a church on the day of my wedding to her father, both of us wearing white. But on this day, as we walked together up the center aisle at Saint Matthew's, we both wore black.

I wore my sunglasses the entire time. I used them to hide my anger and contempt, though everyone else saw a grief-stricken widow-type, since I still had no official title or status, and they didn't know what I knew.

Through the dark shades, I saw everyone as an accomplice to Paulo's charade. Each was a suspect. My internal lens was now clear: no one could be trusted. With each person who approached me, I cringed inside. His family, his friends—had they all known? How could they *not* have known? Why didn't anyone protect me?

TRUTH #1: HIS TRUTH: A REALITY VERY DIFFERENT FROM MINE

After the funeral, our good friends hosted a small reception at their house. A man named Jeff was there.

It hadn't been that long ago when Paulo and I had discussed a recent trip to New York. It had been an odd conversation, one where we danced around Paulo's unclear business dealings, and he had told me to call someone named Jeff if anything happened to him. At the time, I had no idea who Jeff was. At the memorial, I could finally pull him aside and find out what Paulo had meant. In what was meant to be a solemn memorial, I found Jeff right after he had done a few lines of coke in the bathroom.

With a smug sniff as he rubbed the back of his hand against his nose, he said, "I don't know what you're talking about."

Another liar. It was written all over his face, but there was nothing I could do. I had no way of finding out the truth anymore.

I was the girlfriend, the almost-fiancée, of a man caught in a web of women and lies. My jurisdiction was shrinking among his friends, and I was getting shut out, one by one. I wasn't his wife, I wasn't Eden's mom, and my signature wasn't on anything. To all of them, I barely existed, and now I served no further purpose. While I was fading from their view, they all loomed larger in mine. It felt like everyone was complicit in these deceptions. I was determined to find out who had known about Paulo's affairs.

> I was the girlfriend, the almost-fiancée, of a man caught in a web of women and lies.

Paulo had been living in what felt like an alternate universe from the life I thought we'd been sharing together. And I was wrestling to try to piece together these disparate versions of our realities.

When I got back home after the memorial at our friends' place, after slipping into warm pajamas and tumbling into bed, I recalled the Christmas we'd all recently shared at their mountain home in Lake Arrowhead.

On that Christmas morning, we had all gathered by the tree, unwrapping gifts in a round. As Paulo handed me the last gift, I felt everyone holding their breath. I carefully slid my nails under the tape like my grandma taught us back when I was a child and pulled away the paper ever so gently so as not to tear even one corner.

The box showed a picture of a hand blender. *What? Does he want me to learn how to bake?*

But the box seemed too light to be a blender. I opened it and saw another box inside, deep green. It looked familiar and I wasn't quite sure why. But when I pulled out the green box, I saw an emblem I recognized immediately. My dad had collected Rolexes for years. *Is this another trick, or is there really going to be a watch inside?*

Several months earlier, as Paulo and I were making plans to get a rental home together, he'd handed me a jewelry box with an air of anticipation. Catching my breath, expecting to find an engagement ring inside, I was crushed and embarrassed by my excitement to find that the box held a house key. *Fool me once . . .*

So after the key-in-the-velvet-ring-box episode, I opened the Christmas package with less certainty, but there it was: a Rolex with a diamond-encrusted band, white gold shimmering under the mountain-house chandelier. Since Paulo couldn't find the words to express his love, I looked at each diamond like a little beacon of hope. And for him to shower me with that kind of extravagance, I felt valued, worthy, and loved in that moment. All that I had been longing for shimmered on that December night.

We celebrated as a family entering the new year with what seemed like a new sense of *us*. I was convinced this would be the year he'd propose.

Lying in my bed after the memorial and my run-in with Jeff, I was struck by the gap in the truth. How could our realities have been so vastly different? The reality I'd imagined was one in which the man I loved was ready to propose to me.

TRUTH #2: MY TRUTH: A WORLD THAT ONCE FELT SAFE AND LOVING NOW TURNED HOSTILE

One week after Paulo's funeral, I kind of wanted to punch whoever coined the phrase "what a difference a week makes" after the seven days I'd just endured. I was adjusting quickly to these new emotions. Anger became easy for me. I had heard enough stories, speculations, and versions of Paulo's and my life. I remembered a friend telling me she'd witnessed a woman throwing her wineglass at the projector screen during the memorial while it was showing images of his life with Eden and me. The woman screamed, "This was not his life!" My friend said she ran after her and asked her if she was all right. But unlike the others, she didn't stop to introduce herself.

I wore the role of the woman scorned like I'd been made for it. I didn't want to hear condolences anymore, let alone from people who had known about Paulo's betrayals.

It was dusk, and Loretta and I sat in that house of lies in a quiet moment when no one knew what to say, so no one said

> I wore the role of the woman scorned like I'd been made for it.

anything. Suddenly, a black car with tinted windows rolled up to the front of the house. The headlights hit the front room just enough that I knew it was right outside. I threw open the door and screamed, "Come in! Take whatever you want! This was all a sham! This was all bullshit!"

I was able to read the license plate of the black sedan before it sped away. I immediately texted my friend who was a private investigator and asked him to run the plates. But we didn't wait around to find out who this person was. We packed, locked up, and went to stay at a hotel nearby. We didn't feel safe; we had no idea what kind of trouble Paulo had left behind.

TRUTH #3: NO TRUTH: NOTHING MAKES SENSE

Despite the fact I was paying half the rent on our house, our landlord didn't have much sympathy for me. My name was nowhere on paper. He gave me less than a week to find a new place to live. On my salary alone, I didn't have enough money saved up to pay first and last month's rent, plus a deposit. I had put all my extra money into my music.

The Rolex. I could sell the Rolex he gave me for Christmas. I put the watch in its box and asked a friend to get it appraised.

I felt so relieved to at least have something to contribute financially because my friends were uprooting their current lives to help me get through mine. The money from the watch could get me started in a new place. To my knowledge, Paulo had no will, and his life insurance benefits went to Eden, as was only right. As for our land, where we were supposedly building our dream home, I never heard another thing about it. So, when the call came in about the appraisal, I was anxiously waiting to learn what the watch was worth and get some reassurance that I might get through the next couple of months without too much financial stress.

"The Rolex is fake," my friend told me. "I'm sorry, but I'll need two hundred dollars for the appraisal."

I hung up and threw down my phone. I screamed, I punched pillows, and then I laughed so I wouldn't fall apart and cry. There was no more time for tears. Of course the Rolex was fake, just like our entire relationship. Paulo had orchestrated one big charade to keep everyone exactly where he wanted them.

Finding Out It Was All Fake

Imagine an important person in your life—one you had planned on spending the rest of your life with, in sickness and in health—turns out to be a fraud. Rather than being the person you thought loved you, you discover they primarily loved themselves. They had been manipulating the people in their sphere for years—including you. And now imagine this secret is revealed—which all secrets eventually are.

The discovery of betrayal can be dumbfounding, even devastating. The experience can initially include shock, disorientation, and confusion; the lies you were told don't make sense at first. Over time, the experience of betrayal can lead to self-doubt, confusion, and shame. There's a process of looking back over the relationship, scouring memories to see what warning signs you missed. And then there is a process of healing with therapy and self-compassion that can help you move past it.

I've heard this story of waking up to the truth of a narcissistic partner told many different times, but the experience is always overwhelming. One woman described her life with a narcissist like living in a Hollywood movie set for an old cowboy movie. She thought it was real but soon learned it was mostly three-quarter-sized fronts of old buildings. Her life with her partner had been fake, and now she had to reestablish reality and reconnect with people who cared about her.

TRUTH #4: *THE* TRUTH: WAKING UP AND RECOGNIZING THE PEOPLE WHO ARE TRULY ON MY SIDE

When my life went up in flames along with Paulo's plane, my dear friends Shelton and Michelle turned their lives upside down to care for me. They uprooted their lives and offered to find a place with me. I should have gone home to Montana. Away from what had become familiar, I could have forced myself to do the hard work of healing. But I was angry and was going to push that grief into a tiny compartment in my mind. I told myself I was fine. Although I didn't get to see Eden much in that first year, I felt so strongly that I needed to be there for her, or at least close enough where I could get to her at a moment's notice.

Leaving their living situations, uprooting their own lives, the three of us signed a lease together. Shelton and Michelle were my anchors during that stormy season. As I was going through my trauma, they were trauma-adjacent.

In many ways, they went through it too. Living on the Venice canals, we'd canoe the canals and take walks by the ocean. They just listened as I processed, as I remembered, as I raged. I found anger to be an easier place to dwell than sadness. And they were there with me through it all.

At the time I was commuting to Santa Ana to work for Lamar Odom's clothing line, and it could take up to four hours every day to get from our canal house in Venice to Santa Ana and back. I would use that time in the car to talk to myself, give fake interviews, write songs, and sing at the top of my lungs.

> I found anger to be an easier place to dwell than sadness.

I should have taken a grief sabbatical. I should have seen a therapist or gone to a bereavement support group. Instead, I went back to work too soon. I told others what I desperately wanted to believe: "I'm fine." I pushed through. Lamar and his team were patient with my broken heart and accepted my defiant insistence that I was okay.

One day I came home from work to a box sitting outside our front door. It was simply wrapped, with my dad's return address on it. I wasn't expecting anything, but it had a weight to it. I thought it was probably Mace or a Taser since I couldn't have my gun in LA—or maybe bear spray for the wild streets of Venice. As I cut the packing tape with a pair of scissors from the kitchen, I noticed a familiar green color poking out from the slits of the cardboard.

It was an authentic Rolex, heavy and simple. My dad wanted me to look at that watch and be reminded every day that the right man, an honest man, would come along. I prayed that one would.

Real Love and Romance

Real love is often sitting right in front of us, patient, quiet, and steadfast, but romance can lead us to chase excitement and passion. We hope the excitement holds real love, but sometimes it doesn't. As humans, we are wired for love in a conflicting way. We seek commitment and caring and compassion, but we also seek sexual attraction, passion, and desire. Ideally, we want both in a partner, but when we first start a relationship, we're usually looking for the passion and hope the compassion comes later.

Some cultures solve this problem by having arranged marriages. You trust your parents won't set you up with someone who is toxic. The problem with arranged marriages is you end up with a loving person, yet the passion isn't there. In more individualistic societies, we select our mates based on attraction. This is a risky way of doing things because passion isn't as long-lived as compassion.

Similarly, passion and attraction are more enticing in the short term than authentic, compassionate love. So it's natural for us to end up with partners who don't match with us in the long run. It often takes both time and heartbreak to value those authentic, loving relationships.

For further reflection:

- **Notice how each of you is invested in the relationship.** Do you know how and where your partner spends their time? Are you the one who does more things to benefit the relationship in a typical day? Or is your partner the one who carries most of the load?

- **Stay grounded.** What grounds you? Is it being in nature, connecting with God or spirit, being with family, running or athletics, playing music? What are the spaces that keep you in touch with *yourself*?

- **Receive support from others you trust.** When you find yourself disoriented or confused about life or relationships, who can you turn to that you know has your best interests at heart? In other words, who are the rocks in your life? Once you've identified those who will support you when you're feeling down, what is it about them that makes them supportive? How could you add more of these kinds of people in your life?

WHEN YOU'RE OUT OF A TOXIC RELATIONSHIP

I t wasn't until I was out of my toxic relationship that I was able to see it for what it was. But that didn't happen overnight. It took time. It took courage. It took vulnerability. It took the support of the people who loved me.

Maybe, like me, you are finally free of the toxic person to whom you were once bound. But that doesn't mean there's not still work to be done. Once you're out of a toxic relationship, you finally have space to do that work and to heal. You have room to breathe again. You have room to reflect and see what was really going on in your relationship. And I want to encourage you to *keep doing the work*. Give yourself the time and space you deserve to heal.

I encourage you to do this work before entering your next romantic relationship. If you do not take the time to heal, no matter how much you promise yourself you will find someone "better," you'll keep repeating the same old patterns. (I speak with authority. You'll see.)

Getting out of the relationship is your first step toward freedom. Now keep going.

6

GRIEVING THE
LOST YEARS

*How We Deal (or
Don't) with the Loss*

Somehow, I made it to the one-year anniversary of
Paulo's death.

By that point, I'd decided this milestone would sig-
nify my personal renaissance. It would be my rebirth. Like a
phoenix, I was rising from the ashes and choosing *me* for the
first time in I don't know how long. I had a lot of time to make
up for, not to mention the fear of running out of time. The time
was now. I wasn't going to let anyone or anything get in my way.

I just didn't know that *I* was the one who was in my own way. During that first year especially, I had developed some coping strategies along the way.

COPING STRATEGY #1: WE DISTRACT OURSELVES PROFESSIONALLY

Back home in Montana, I found myself in an unexpected conversation about losing a loved one, grief, and the healing power of music.

A local family in my hometown had lost their son, a Marine killed in combat in Afghanistan. The stories were devastating, and I could relate to that sickening feeling of immediate, life-changing tragedy. As I offered my sympathies and shared my personal experience and comprehension of tragedy, the father humbly stated that he had written a poem. He asked if I would consider reworking it into a song. This wasn't unheard of; I had written songs for individuals and organizations before. And how could I say no to a grieving family? I wished them well and said that I would keep in touch and share the work once I had written and arranged it.

Several weeks later, I sat cross-legged on the floor of their living room with my guitar and sang into their hearts. I poured out my own broken heart through a poem a father had written for his fallen son. That night changed the course of the entire year for me.

They were so moved that we scheduled to record it with my producer, Jim, in LA mid-January. Soon after the song was finished, Bob, the bereaved dad, started securing opportunities for me to perform for Gold Star Families on Marine bases across the country, as well as on aircraft carriers during Fleet Week, all leading up to a fifty-date Military Appreciation Tour. This was backed by a major multi-level marketing (MLM) company along with a contract to be the face of their cosmetic brand.

I was more than happy to lose myself in my work.

In fact, it felt like the whole world was aligning in my favor. Finally, here was my chance. Maybe there was a reason I'd had to suffer so much. I was finally going to be able to make ends meet financially through my music. Things seemed to be coming together in the most extraordinary way, as if they had

> I was more than happy to lose myself in my work.

God written all over them. It felt like the perfect storm of giving back, living my purpose, and building my business.

Who could I call in the business to help make this possible? I had to plan for touring and all the things that followed. Danny, Dolly Parton's manager, came to mind. He was an acquaintance through a mutual friend in LA. He would know what to do. He kept things simple and to the point. "Once everything is signed, sealed, and delivered, I can absolutely help. Keep me posted," Danny said. So that is exactly what I did.

The contract had been overseen by my attorney, one of the most respected entertainment lawyers in the business, papers had been signed, and I was set to fly to Michigan to meet with the entire team that summer. We were ready. After watching this song and the intensity of our stories coming together, I could see healing happen from the stage.

While planning was taking place for the Military Appreciation Tour with the MLM company, Bob set up small performances across the country. I performed at modest events on military bases and for the Gold Star Families. I felt as if I were a vessel, and this was what my voice was made for. Of course, I wanted the platinum records, sold-out tours, and all the things that come with that, but this was special. I was helping people through their most devastating losses, even while I was working through mine.

Having traveled to Ada, Michigan, to meet the team from the MLM, I was waiting in my hotel room when Bob called to say that their biggest Chinese distributor had unexpectedly come to town; we would have to reschedule this initial signing meeting. I was disappointed, but my positivity overrode my gut feeling that something was off. "This is only a minor setback," I told myself. "The contract is signed; everything will come together. It's just a matter of time."

But days turned into months. And while I'd assumed Bob was working hard to get everything sorted with our sponsors, the holidays came and went, and after calls, texts, and emails, the response was still silence. Bob had gone AWOL. I searched the internet and found the number for the MLM. I immediately got to the person I needed to speak with. She said she was so happy to hear from me. She wondered what had happened as they were so excited to do an appreciation concert for the military base. *One concert?* It was a gut punch—not fifty, just one, and I was not going to be the face of anything.

A few months later, I received an unexpected call from Bob's wife. The conversation led to her sharing and exposing more than I could have ever seen coming about her now soon-to-be ex. In addition to their house burning down, losing everything, and being left destitute, Bob's wife said he had told her we were having an affair. *Respectfully, no.* Bob had left her and their kids with nothing. He had used his son's tragic death to use people, to work them over, and he is still on the run to this day.

It turned out everything had been a lie, all over again, but this time it was in my professional life. Bob had cost me money, time, and my reputation.

> It turned out everything had been a lie, all over again.

All I had left was debt and damage control to be managed on my own. I was sitting in disbelief and shame—again.

Distracting Ourselves with Work

When we experience a powerful emotional shock, such as from a romantic betrayal, the immediate results include disorientation and psychological pain. It's normal to feel confused and out of control.

One very human response to those feelings is to try to regain control of our lives. How do we do that? Well, if we love our job and we're good at it, a natural thing to do is throw ourselves into our work. This isn't something everyone does; often, the last thing people want to do after a major psychological blow is go back to work. But for people who feel professionally competent and receive positive feedback on their accomplishments, doubling down on work makes sense. It can lead to a sense of control and euphoria. However, if the psychological work hasn't been done to understand the trauma and to work through some of the emotional pain, there is a risk of falling into the same relationship pattern again with another toxic partner.

It's important to remember that trauma needs to be understood, and often the pain needs to be re-experienced before a person can move forward in a healthy way. This inner work can be painful and lonely, whereas outer work can be exciting and lead to receiving praise from outsiders. Although there is nothing wrong with getting back to work to gain some self-confidence after a bad breakup, it's also important to take some time and work through the emotional pain of the experience.

COPING STRATEGY #2: WE DISTRACT OURSELVES PERSONALLY

As the summer approached, six months after the crash, my strength began increasing. I started eating again. My friends said it was time for me to be in a public setting as a single woman. This seemed like a terrible idea. I felt far from ready. But I conceded and put my best, most awkward foot forward—and directly into my mouth. As we stood at a dimly lit Beverly Hills bar, an unassuming guy in his mid-thirties approached me and started up a conversation. His looks were striking, and he spoke with both kindness and directness. Noticing I wasn't wearing a ring, he asked if I had a boyfriend.

Do I? I suddenly had no idea. I had been trying to figure out my identity as this quasi widow, but there's no word for what I was.

In that moment, I heard myself utter a strange, incomplete sentence I never imagined compiling to this nice man: "I have a dead."

There was no second sentence. That was all of it.

No doubt startled and confused, he walked away. I busted out laughing for probably the first time since the crash. Glancing at my friends' faces, I could tell exactly what they were thinking: *Oh, shit! She's not ready for the outside yet. Get her back inside.*

> I had been trying to figure out my identity as this quasi widow, but there's no word for what I was.

Mortified, they rushed me out of the bar and didn't attempt another such adventure again for some time. I laughed all the way home.

Not long after, I got into a relationship with a man I'll simply refer to as "the Prince." He was worldly, cultured, and had lived in Europe and spoke French, even though he had been born and raised in California. He was my first relationship after Paulo's death.

One evening I was having dinner with my girlfriend Brandi. She asked about the Prince, who was in Switzerland at the moment, where he lived and worked most of the time.

When I reported that I thought we were doing well, her demeanor changed in front of my eyes. Brandi admitted she was hoping I'd say I had broken things off with him. She told me one of her friends had recently hooked up with him in the back of her car after giving him a ride home. After their encounter, he'd threatened to destroy her if she told anyone because he had a girlfriend.

I turned every shade of shame, hurt, anger, and betrayal. *How am I in this position again?* I had just navigated the lies in my business and come out the other side.

The words the Prince had gently spoken to me not long after we met rang in my ears, *I'm going to show you that you can trust men again.*

Seriously, I can't make this shit up.

"Attention, shoppers! The Quayle has a bad case of repeater syndrome."

REPETITION COMPULSION: This behavior involves repeating painful situations that occurred in the past. It's a way to ease tension from physical or emotional trauma, but it doesn't always work that way. This unconscious "trauma reenactment" can include any experience where you feel overwhelmed with hopelessness or fear.[2]

I thanked my friend for her friendship and for her honesty. I begged her to tell me who the woman was. She said she couldn't tell me, that she had promised her friend anonymity.

At the time, I was living with a friend outside of Nashville, Tennessee, in a city called Franklin. On my way home, I wanted to drive off the road. Gripping the wheel, I called my stepmom. I wish I could tell you she was surprised, but she wasn't. My roommate had gone out of town, and I was alone in her house in a devastated state of mind. I got out a handle of vodka and drank until my fingers dialed the Prince's Swiss number.

"I can't hurt anymore," I announced when I heard his voice. "I'm done."

And then I hung up.

The Prince called Brandi, who showed up at the house with a suicide prevention counselor from Vanderbilt University Medical Center. After spending time speaking with me, they agreed to let me sleep off the alcohol, and Brandi kindly stayed by my side.

The next morning I went to the kitchen to fix myself some breakfast, and as I reached for a knife, it broke my heart to see the knives had been placed on the highest shelf so I couldn't hurt myself. I felt disgusted. I was disappointed that I had allowed this to happen again, that I had mistrusted my gut feelings. I'd let the Prince treat me the same way I had been treated by Paulo. I let him convince me I was the problem.

The shame felt even heavier this time. I knew I needed to work on *me*. I was going to get to the bottom of what was going on with me. *I was worth saving.* I was thirty-three at the time.

My family was familiar with an inpatient mental health facility in Aurora, Colorado, where I enrolled in a weeklong program. It was truly a life-changing experience. One of the most vivid moments happened at the end of the week. Along a long line stretching out across a whiteboard, they had me tick off thirty-three marks for each year of my life. And then above the line I wrote down everything good that I could remember: getting my first horse, going to Switzerland for an exchange program, graduating high school. Below the line, I recorded everything not-so-good that had happened in my life: my parents' divorces, being bullied at school, and so on. After I'd completed the exercise, the therapist handed me an eraser and asked me to erase all of it—the good and not-so-good.

While I was making strides, struggling to get free and heal, the Prince wouldn't let me go without a fight. He launched a persuasion campaign that was an

My issues were deep-rooted, and there would be more questions before there were any answers.

all-out assault on my emotions, using every tactic from denial to anger to love bombing to reassurance. He even went as far as asking me to marry him post-breakup.

I discovered my issues were deep-rooted, and there would be more questions before there were any answers. Part of me was still deluded: I was sure I was the problem and that what had been told to me about the Prince and his infidelity was just a jealous woman trying to hurt me.

We stayed together. We even rented a place together, and I continued to find myself in that darker place of "I'm the problem." Some of my friends wondered if I stayed because being with him shielded me from everyone else, or because the pattern of dysfunction felt familiar. I may not have been in the driver's seat, but at least I wasn't in the trunk. My dad and my friends all begged me to see what I couldn't. *Why can't I see clearly? What is wrong with me?*

I may not have been in the driver's seat, but at least I wasn't in the trunk.

What about you? What have your subsequent relationships been like after a toxic one? Sometimes we instinctively jump back into the same kind of mess. Or we might protect ourselves by avoiding relationships altogether. Other times, though, we choose to do the hard work of healing. (Don't worry; I'm getting there! You will too.)

From One Bad Relationship to the Next

After a relationship is over, why do we make the same mistakes again? Why do we find the same bad guy again? Why is it so hard to break the toxic cycle?

You didn't just develop your patterns in relationships last month or last year; you've been learning these patterns since before you were born. Your earliest connections with your parents and other caregivers form the basis of your entire system of attachment to other people. As you grow older your models of relationships become more complex. When you start dating, you often select a certain type of person who comes with a certain relationship pattern. These early loves shape what you look for later, and these patterns tend to be consistent over time.

So when a relationship ends, the most natural thing to do is to find a similar one. If you were in a toxic relationship, you aren't necessarily looking for somebody who is toxic like your partner was. But you still might be looking for the charming and attractive but toxic qualities you fell in love with before you knew how toxic they were.

One way to break the cycle is through insight and self-awareness. If you can study the patterns of your own relationships and start to see how you do the same thing over and over, that can sometimes snap you out of it. Another way to break the cycle is through behavior. Try a different way to meet people. Ask your friends to set you up with someone who seems like a good person. Or maybe go on a few dates with someone you're not super attracted to physically but who has a reputation as a trustworthy individual.

To break your cycle of bad relationships, you need to first identify your pattern and then understand it. Then, you must take active steps to avoid falling into the pattern again. This will likely mean trying some new things that could end up with better results.

COPING STRATEGY #3: WE DO THE HARD WORK OF GRIEVING OUR LOSS

It turns out there was a third way. I didn't *have* to numb myself with work. I didn't *have* to avoid my feelings by jumping into another relationship. That third option, though, wasn't one that interested me at the time.

I know now I could've paused longer to look at what was going on inside me. I could've found a grief counselor, a therapist, a support group—anyone who could have helped me with my loss, with my grief, with my anger. There were so many available resources I simply didn't know about or wasn't ready for. I could have been honest with friends and family about what I'd been through. If I could do it all over, I would have been much more intentional about seeking help.

Today, I'm committed to inner work. Today, I know that the healing journey is one that continues. I'm convinced we must keep choosing it, day after day, making healing a habit.

I wonder what your journey from bondage to freedom has looked like. Have you, like me, found distractions that have kept you from pausing to look inside yourself? Or have you done the hard things? Have you taken baby step after baby step in pursuit of the healing you need and deserve? Wherever you are on your journey today, I encourage you to take the next step.

Doing the Work to Heal

People talk about doing "the work" in healing, but what exactly does that mean? It's the tough, sometimes painful, but ultimately rewarding journey of understanding, emotionally processing, and moving past the trauma of betrayal. Often the work involves looking further into the past to find the sources of more negative relationship patterns. It can involve turning inward, reexperiencing the emotional pain and trauma that might be in your past or gaining insight into your behavioral patterns and habits and how they help you and hurt you, coupled with active efforts to use this new wisdom to be authentically and positively engaged in the real world.

Part of doing the work involves emotionally painful honesty and introspection; the other part involves growing in your current life. In a sense, doing the work is like cleaning out your messy car filled with bad memories and fast-food wrappers until it feels good to drive in again—then taking off in a new and better direction. The work isn't about getting stuck in the past but clearing it so you can move more optimistically into the future.

Here are a few good places to start:

- Seek out a licensed psychotherapist, counselor, or life coach to get a new perspective.
- Read self-help books or spiritual books.

- Try physical or somatic work with your body, like yoga or therapeutic massages.
- Clean up your diet or improve your physical fitness.
- Journal or keep a diary to process and reflect.
- Try a spiritual practice, like meditation or prayer, to help calm the nervous system and reduce that fight-or-flight response.

Sometimes the work can involve getting out of your comfort zone and trying something new, such as an art class or traveling or trying a new church. It's important that the work isn't just something that goes on in your head but something that's expressed in your real life.

For further reflection:

- **Identify the patterns in your relationships.** Do you find yourself dating the same person over and over again? Looking at your past relationships, do you notice any consistent negative behavioral patterns across partners? Do you think your friends notice any negative patterns in your behavior? If yes, when do you think those started?

- **Consider your relationship to your work.** In your job, do you feel positively connected and experience deep engagement? Do you ever lose yourself in your work in a healthy way? Do you feel that you're a bit of a workaholic? Reflect on the things you do that bring you authentic joy at work. How could you do more of those?

- **Notice how you do or don't blame others.** Do you blame others for your unhealthy patterns and choices? How could you take more responsibility for doing the work and improving yourself without the intense and negative emotions of shame?

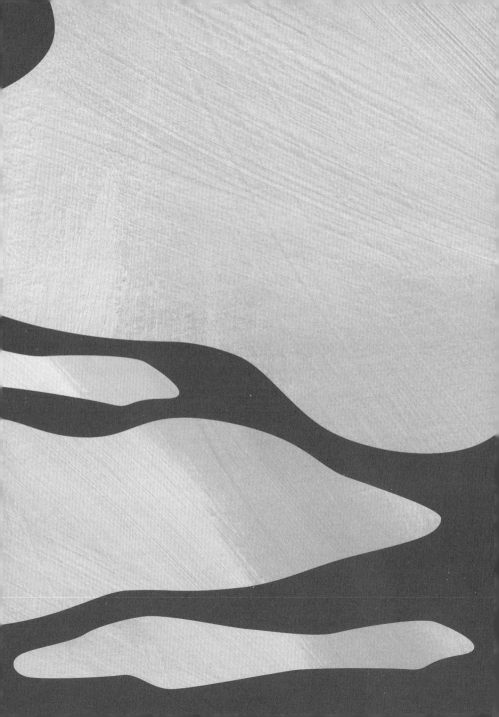

7

RIPPLE EFFECTS

> *How We Stop the Cycle and*
> *Prepare for Something Better*

After Paulo's death, I kept myself busy with my work. I hustled to write songs, record songs, and get gigs. I wrote about everything except for what I should have written about—the grief and the lost years. I got tangled up in another unhealthy romantic relationship, and I got burned by a toxic business relationship. Through it all, I assured everyone

I was fine, and on my good days even believed it was true. I avoided looking at my pain until I could no longer outrun it. Eventually I reached a point where I needed to face my trauma head-on and stop the cycle.

WAY TO STOP THE CYCLE #1: DO THE WORK

Finally, on the recommendation of one of my friends, I signed up for one-on-one grief counseling at Alive Hospice in Nashville. Within a few weeks, I heard about the group therapy sessions but found out I wasn't eligible. Essentially, my grief had "aged out" because the group sessions were for those who had lost someone within the previous six months. I pleaded my case, saying I'd be an example of what *not* to do after a tragic loss of a loved one, and eventually the committee allowed me to join the group.

In that group setting I learned I wasn't alone and that everything I was feeling in the grief department was standard issue. It was such a strange camaraderie of humans who'd lost loved ones to cancer and car accidents and heart disease and, in my case, a plane crash. It was this caring, tight-knit club that no one chose to be in, yet everyone was grateful to be a part of. I discovered that every cliché has a place and time. I learned grief can be an enemy or a friend, but it won't disappear and will even find you when you think you have outrun it—but you simply can't outrun it.

On the last day of the course, our group leader asked what the one thing was—if there was one thing—to take away from this time together. I found myself saying out loud to the group of first-name-only friends, "I will no longer be held hostage by these chains of grief."

The Healing Journey

When you begin your journey toward healing, it's useful to have good resources that can help you navigate the path, such as other people who have been on your same journey or who have good knowledge of the journey. These might be friends or family, specific support groups, a wise mentor or spiritual counselor, a licensed psychotherapist or psychologist, or even a coach, MD, or attorney. Surrounding yourself with good people who know what's going on and have your best interests at heart is crucial for moving forward. It's hard to do it alone.

Also consider surrounding yourself with a healthy environment. For example, being outdoors in nature can be very healing,[3] so it might be useful to spend time outdoors in beautiful areas. I also suggest keeping your physical health strong. Exercise can boost confidence and buffer depression. People who eat a lot of nutrient-dense foods report less depression and greater levels of happiness and mental well-being.[4] Healthy food will increase your energy level. Our minds, bodies, and relationships are all tied up together in a system, and the healthier we are physically, the healthier we will be mentally.[5]

A major part of healing is growing psychologically. So, when you are in the process of grieving and healing, take some time for soul-searching. Travel, read nonfiction literature, listen to music, and try some new things. It's important to work through the trauma of betrayal, but there is also a risk of getting trapped in self-analysis— what people sometimes call "analysis paralysis"—so keep engaging in the world and look for the joy.

The work of looking inward and healing is challenging but worth it. This process will be easier if you surround yourself with people who can help you on your journey. And it will be even easier if you surround yourself with a healthy environment.

WAY TO STOP THE CYCLE #2: FACE THE TRUTH

I'm not proud of it today, but I stayed with the Prince longer than I should have.

While the Prince was still politicking me to stay with him, I found the courage to track down the girl who had accused him, and I begged her to meet me for coffee at Frothy Monkey in Nashville. When we met, I could tell she was mortified to have agreed to this. I could feel her shame as soon as I walked in the door. I promised I wasn't mad at her and said I would never tell anyone who she was.

What mattered most, I assured her, was that she was the key to my being able to walk away.

I began by sharing my traumatic past with her and why I was seeking her counsel.

"I'm not capable in this moment to leave," I admitted. "My compass is broken. I'm all jacked up. Will you please just tell me what he said to you?"

I had to know the truth.

While much of what she told me tracked as being true, including the kind of protection he used, the final detail she reported is what sealed the deal.

When they hooked up, she hadn't been aware that he was in a relationship. But at the close of the evening, he threatened her: "If you tell anyone, I'll destroy your career."

That's when I knew. The tone in which she repeated it rang true to something within me. I recognized her fear.

He was a bully, and that was the exact language I'd heard him use when he was on business calls.

She was telling the truth. It was the Prince who was the liar.

Even though I knew the truth, I still didn't leave him after my conversation with this girl.

The final, *final* straw (I know, that's a lot of straws—the box is almost empty) happened soon after, when we were in Cabo, Mexico, celebrating his birthday.

We were at the beach, and I'd grabbed his phone to take a picture of us. When I peeked to see if it had been a good shot, I found countless explicit photos of women on his camera roll.

His excuse?

"I look at these pictures so I don't cheat on you."

Damn, he was good.

We somehow took our argument from the beachfront to the hotel restaurant and ended up leaving the restaurant abruptly when we got louder than the music. Our intense conversation continued until we were back in our hotel room. As we argued, he was lying on the bed and I was standing in front of the television. He got so angry at my accusations that he picked up the television remote and threw it toward me. Missing me, it shattered the television screen.

That night I slept outside on beach chairs, wrapped in beach towels and surrounded by empty mini alcohol bottles I had downed to find comfort.

When we checked out the next morning, he calmly reported to the desk staff that he'd slipped on the tile in the room, hitting the television with his elbow, and since it was their tile that was slippery, he shouldn't be held responsible for the damages. He was so convincing I found myself believing him too, even though only hours before I'd watched the TV remote fly through the air, the TV taking the hit instead of my face.

Having been rattled by the woman who'd exposed his infidelity, I had been looking for apartments before we went to Mexico for his birthday. When I got back, I worked stealthily so I could get myself moved to my own place while he was out of the country.

The Courage It Takes to Face the Truth

It's easy to follow the path you're already on; this is the power of inertia. Even if we're on a bad path, it's one that's familiar to us and, in a strange way, we might feel comfortable there. If you're dating a toxic person, for example, the relationship will have awful aspects, but it also has a friendship network, social status, and the chance it might improve. Leaving and starting a new path is scary, and there are no guarantees.

Because change is so difficult, it can take some work to get it kickstarted. You might need a jolt. In Alcoholics Anonymous (AA), there is a saying about hitting "rock bottom." Many people don't stop drinking until it becomes so bad they simply must stop. Jail time from a DUI or losing a job will certainly lead a person to rock bottom.

The other thing we need is the courage to face the truth of the situation; we need to be honest about how toxic the situation is. We need to admit to ourselves that we made a mistake, accept that we must cut our losses, and then leave the relationship. And then we need to be willing to face the unknown—the anger or bitterness, and the possible feelings of loneliness when we are by ourselves again, along with the challenge of building a new life.

We will naturally resist change until some outside force or experience jolts us awake. It will require courage and honesty to begin the best path forward.

WAY TO STOP THE CYCLE
#3: MAKE THE BREAK

I was finally able to leave the Prince with the full conviction of not only his infidelity but his ability to lie, which he did with such ease it scared me. While he was in Switzerland, I packed up everything of mine in the apartment we shared. There was no trace of me left when he came back. I had to leave in this way so he couldn't put another spell on me. He *wasn't* the one to show me I could trust men again. If anything, he reinforced my distrust.

I moved to a one-bedroom apartment in a secured building, just me and Mijo, my Chihuahua mix that Eden and I had adopted off the streets of Venice Beach years earlier, and a mattress on the floor. For months to come, the Prince would try to convince me to come back to him, but I didn't back down. I had more courage to fight for myself than I'd ever had before. Eventually, the calls and orchids stopped arriving, and he stopped trying to convince my family to intercede. It was over. This time I'd had the strength to leave.

But I had lost years.

The Courage It Takes to Leave

Leaving your current life and embarking on a journey to an unknown future that you hope is better takes enormous courage. Courage doesn't always come easy, which is why we honor and celebrate heroes, retelling their stories for millennia. But great heroes relied on allies and cleverness as much as boldness to beat a greater foe. So when you're reaching inward for the courage to leave a bad relationship, also reach outward to friends or mentors.

If you are ready to leave a bad relationship, you don't need to have a face-to-face blowup or fight with your toxic partner; you can just leave. One of my favorite pieces of advice for exiting a toxic relationship is simple: "Rent a U-Haul. Leave a note." A toxic relationship doesn't need to be solved; it needs to be ended. What needs to be solved are the psychological and social forces that keep pushing you toward toxic relationships, and that can only be done when you are out of the toxic relationship you're in. Be strong—and also be smart and keep yourself safe.

WAY TO STOP THE CYCLE #4:
CHOOSE WHAT'S GOOD

On a trip to North Carolina to perform at a show for the Commissioner of Agriculture for the state of North Carolina, I met Jason. He was the representative from the event and we met at a corner booth in Elizabeth's Pizza in Greensboro, where he introduced me to someone named David Couch, one of the event sponsors. David was forty-five minutes late; he'd been in a fender bender.

At the time, I was still dating the Prince. All I knew was I wanted to hide out in the happiness of this weekend's performance and a room full of strangers who were unaware of how close I had come to losing my life just weeks prior. Here, I could hide in my songs and my smile and my personality. I could be whomever I wanted to be. And in this moment, I was a country singer from Nashville set to headline a big event. Nice to meet you!

> All I knew was I wanted to hide out in the happiness of this weekend's performance.

David was handsome and kind. He thanked me for coming out and said he hoped I would like the cozy accommodations of the little cabin on his farm, Summerfield Farms. On Sunday, he drove me to catch my flight, but on our way, we stopped at a restaurant near the airport for breakfast.

Over breakfast, David innocently asked, "So where you headed?"

"Well," I began in earnest, "my boyfriend has been accused of cheating on me. But I don't believe it. He would never do that." At that time I couldn't imagine the Prince ever doing something so horrible, especially after knowing everything I had gone through with Paulo.

Feeling like David deserved more information, I continued, "I had a really bad night—drank a lot of vodka—and I'm putting myself in emotional rehab in Colorado because I have a bad picker."

Sitting back, David considered what I'd offered.

Kindly, he clarified, "I meant where are you traveling to today?"

Of course he did.

I continued to spill my entire life story to this Southern gentleman, who listened to much more than he'd asked for.

When we said our goodbyes at the airport in Greensboro, he said, "Good on you for doing this work. Let me know what happens."

David would definitely find out what happened.

For further reflection:

- **Consider seeking support from a group.** For some of us, reaching out to a support group, in our town or online, is second nature. For others, it can feel uncomfortable to reach out. If you have tried this, what benefits did you experience? Have you looked into group support? If not, then why?

- **Name a time you exercised courage.** Maybe you faced a physical threat like a bear, or a dangerous person, or even a crazy amusement park ride. What gave you the strength to be courageous? Was it something you felt inside, or was it just your automatic response to the threat? Sometimes courage comes before we have a chance to get scared or talk ourselves out of it.

- **Notice who you support.** Sometimes we help ourselves through helping others. Across a wide body of psychological research, we see that being kind and helping others can boost our own sense of joy, connection, and well-being.[6] How are you supporting others now? Brainstorm some opportunities where you could help other people.

8

BEGINNING TO LIVE AGAIN

How We Overcome the Past

December in Montana was like a dream. For me, *any* month in Montana is like a dream. But this trip home would be one that would change my armored heart's course forever.

PATH #1: BE OPEN TO NEW POSSIBILITIES

I'd been presenting an annual concert for the food bank in my hometown of Bozeman, and it was that time of year again.

Usually, I would arrive home a few days earlier than the show date to do press and promotions and get the word out the best I knew how, with my own words, face-to-face, to build excitement about what we were planning to do for our community.

David—the guy I'd met in North Carolina—and I had stayed in touch that year. We'd occasionally catch up on each other's lives, and I'd hear about his world, and he'd hear about mine. After the weeklong rehab program, though, I called David to share how great it had been. In addition to learning more about me, he was fascinated by the music industry and how different it was from his business of real estate development and ranching. I shared the highs and lows of the business and the touring lifestyle I was living, all the while navigating therapy, grief counseling, and trying to rid myself of the sticky web of lies from my previous relationship with Paulo.

David shared with me that his son, Andrew, who lived in North Carolina, wanted to go to outfitters school outside of Bozeman and learn to take horses and mules into the mountains with camping gear to accompany people who wanted to stay on the land.

"Heads up," I warned. "If you go to Montana, you're going to fall in love with it. Just know that going in; it will take ahold of your heart."

Some time went on and I continued trying to put my life back together, which included breaking up with the Prince.

David had been considering taking a monthlong sabbatical from work, and he decided to spend a month out west while Andrew was in Montana. Although he'd planned to drive through Idaho and Wyoming, the valley he fell in love with was forty-five minutes from my hometown. (Weird-but-true story: He'd seen a Montana house in a magazine and had always wanted to buy land and build a house like the one he'd seen. When he hunted it down, the actual house from the magazine was *for sale*. Crazy, right? And yeah, he bought it.)

Our worlds became serendipitously closer throughout David's time in Montana.

One afternoon late in December, before he was heading back to North Carolina, David offered, "Why don't you come out and see the place?"

He let me know that he wouldn't be able to stay for the benefit concert as he had to get home to celebrate the holidays with his kids. When I got off the phone to make my way to visit him, something was different. I was nervous. I put on my go-to light-gray turtleneck. (I'm known for my hives when I'm nervous and I could already feel them populating my chest like an unwelcome guest.) I felt like a teenager as I borrowed my dad's car to drive to Emigrant, Montana. Steam was rising from the Yellowstone River to my left as I drove

> Our worlds became serendipitously closer.

through Paradise Valley. Keith Urban's song "We Were Us" was playing on the radio, and I was speeding along the two lanes to the unknown.

When I pulled up the circular driveway covered in snow, I stepped out of the car in my boots and jeans to see David standing in the open doorway of his home.

Before I could even say hello, he gestured inside and said, "Welcome home."

Is this really happening?

It hadn't been in the realm of possibility that he could be interested in me. I don't get the good guy. I get the other guys.

I was guarded, but there was something about him that felt like home.

It's no surprise survivors of abuse from narcissistic partners pull from the lessons of our past, is it? I believe there was some reason I was in a toxic relationship, or in my case *relationships*, in the first place. But once we learn our behavioral patterns and obtain some healing and self-love, we owe it to ourselves to be wise about the relationships that come next.

> We owe it to ourselves to be wise about the relationships that come next.

Making the Next One a Good One

Moving on from a toxic relationship into a new romance is challenging. How do we know we're not going to end up in the same place we did before? There's no single answer, but there are strategies you can use that will boost your confidence in making better decisions moving forward with a new partner.

Step back and look at the new partner's relationship history. Instead of rushing in, wade in and do some serious homework along the way. If the new partner is a good prospect, they will have lived a good life. This doesn't mean they're perfect or don't have a past; it means there will be plenty of evidence of warm and loving relationships across their life. They will have a group of friends and family whom they treat with respect and who respect them. They will get along with people at work and in the world. They will have a good reputation for treating people fairly and ethically. Don't fall headlong into love with a man of mystery; instead, "fall in like" with a person who, by all accounts, seems to be of high moral character, work ethic, and affection.

Listen to the feedback of your friends, family, advisors, and other people you trust. If everybody is getting a bad vibe or knows provable negative information about your new love interest, those people are probably a better indicator of the future of your relationship than your current feelings of infatuation—however enjoyable and powerful they might be.

Finally, look for changes in yourself. If you've done the work after your past toxic relationship and have grown as a person, you should notice this in your own initial attraction and romance. You're being a little wiser. You're not rushing into things. You also might be feeling deeper connections beyond the initial butterflies of new romance. You might notice that your life outside the relationship is getting better as you get deeper in the relationship. If the fruits of your relationship are you becoming a better person, that's a good sign.

There's always a risk when you start a new relationship. But if you do the work of psychological healing, and you're smart and deliberate in your decisions, your chances of getting hurt are going to go way down.

PATH #2: RESIST THE OLD PATTERNS

David and I talked for hours. I won't lie; I had feelings for him. Feelings of hope paired with sabotaging self-talk. My inner voice told me, *Don't get ahead of yourself. You don't get the good guy.*

I remember as a child I had a powerful dream of a black piano next to windows overlooking water—not a lake or a pond but moving water. And in David's living room I saw a black piano against these windows that overlooked a flowing stream on his property.

As I walked across the living room, a photo of his daughter caught my eye. The thought that went through my head in that instant was, *We could be close one day.* Immediately, there was a voice tempering expectations. *You're getting ahead of yourself, Quayle; rein it in.* As David and I sat on his black leather couch, hours flew by as we enjoyed our captivating conversation.

Here's the thing, though: I knew I was still fragile. I knew I should not be allowed to make any decision in the department of love. And yet these feelings were undeniable. In two words: *raging pheromones.* I knew I had to leave before we crossed any lines.

So I popped up suddenly and announced, "I must leave."

He laughed at me, walked me to the door, and kissed my forehead. I drove home feeling like a teenage girl, and my parents knew when I walked through the doors that I was a smitten kitten.

David came back after Christmas, and by January, you couldn't keep us apart. We were inseparable in our impenetrable love bubble. We had an ease about us. With him, it was unnecessary to be anything but myself, in all my flawed glory. I didn't have to try like I did in previous relationships. All my "try" had gone up in flames, and that was a good thing. David saw me, loved me, and wanted me just as I was, as I am. Plus, he was already aware of all my stuff from when I shared it the first time we sat down, just the two of us. I wasn't broken to him, just a great work of art in progress. *If only you could see yourself the way I see you,* he'd said.

We both came to the relationship with our pasts, but our present overshadowed them in bright, loving light. He was patient and kind, and I was all his. Somehow the heart I had cordoned off in metal sheets and carefully welded together had gotten bit hard by love. But this love felt different; it felt holy.

I wanted to be sure not to make the same mistakes I'd made in the past.

Doing Things Differently from the Start

If what you've done in the past hasn't worked when starting a new relationship, it's important to change things up a bit. The first and foremost strategy I suggest to people in these situations is to *go slow*! There is no need to rush into a brand-new relationship. It's better to walk into the right relationship that will be there for the long term. So take your time and get to know the person and do your homework on them.

The second thing I suggest is to consider going against your heart or gut at times. Let me be clear: If your gut is telling you this is a dangerous or a shady individual, then trust your gut and get away immediately. But if you're not having immediate romantic feelings for a potential partner, but you enjoy being around the person and they have a lot of great qualities, consider overriding your initial reaction and give the person a chance. It doesn't mean it's going to work out, but since your heart has put you with some toxic characters in the past, maybe let yourself be driven a little more by your head and see how that works.

The final suggestion I have is to get outside of your comfort zone a little bit. If up until now you've been meeting people in a certain place or in a certain industry, and your results have been less than impressive, it might be time to shake things up.

PATH #3: SAY YES TO WHAT'S BEST

When David took me up on a hill in Montana, it was a day like any other day. I was in my camo hat, jeans, and boots. We were planning on going four-wheeling, which was not unusual at all. As we got situated in our spot on top of the hillside overlooking beautiful Paradise Valley, his buddy Church was texting me about some details for his and David's upcoming trip.

"Will you put down your phone?" David said abruptly.

"It's not like I'm on social media," I said. "It's your friend Church asking about shotgun shells."

He followed that with, "But you said all I had to do was take you up on a hill in Montana and ask you to marry me."

Wait, what?

A few months earlier, we'd committed to the idea of spending our lives together. I assured him that I did not need any kind of fancy proposal. "Just take me up on a hill in Montana and ask me to marry you," I joyfully instructed. "I don't need anything fancy. All I want is you."

As he slipped the ring on my finger, a jolt sprang into my step, and I started screaming from the tops of my lungs, "We're engaged! We're engaged!" followed by running myself out of breath back into his arms in awe of his love for me and my love for him. He was so calm, I wondered what he was feeling inside. He sure didn't show his hand at all. If he was nervous, it was hidden behind his loving blue eyes. We were combining our lives, including his kids, their mom, his career, my career, and my touring the country. Everything was moving fast, and every moment was momentous. It felt like the past had finally lost its hold on me and love had conquered all.

After a toxic relationship ends, we want to do things differently. We want to get it right. But I didn't want to give up on the one thing I had always wanted: love.

For me, saying yes to a healthy relationship was right. But for someone else, the right thing may be to take a break from relationships altogether. For someone else, the right thing might be going back to school, or it might be saying yes to a new job. As we begin to live well, we say yes to what nourishes and strengthens us.

> I didn't want to give up on the one thing I had always wanted: love.

The Courage to Say Yes

Saying yes to life shows a massive display of courage. It could mean saying yes to another romantic relationship, but it doesn't have to. Perhaps you've realized it's best to stay out of romantic relationships for a while so you can put your energy toward a creative or philanthropic project, your personal growth, health, or fitness. Or you might want to spend more time with your family or a friend group. Maybe you want to work on your spiritual growth. There is no right answer to life, but the wrong answer is to live in fear and cut yourself off from any opportunity for growth.

No matter what choice you make, there is always risk when you embrace life. There is a risk in love because of rejection and loss. Even if you find true and lasting love, it can be lost someday, even for natural reasons.

But here are some suggestions for getting out there and saying yes. Start small but be consistent. You don't need to make dramatic changes; focus on making small changes in a consistent way. Consider different activities that you could do regularly with friends—maybe a daily walk, a creative project, working out, or attending social events—anything that calls to you. Over time you'll become more engaged, self-confident, and hopefully connected to the social world and your physical body. That new strength and social connection will allow you to say yes to even more things in life. Growth will start compounding and accelerating. In time, maybe a year or two in the future, as you continue to look back at your past self, you'll notice the changes. You'll see just how far you've come.

PATH #4: REFUSE TO IGNORE THE HURTING PLACES

The thing about the past is that it's always near.

Even though I now had a wonderful man in my life, I was still undone. Still living in a lot of shame.

I had this man who was telling me he loved me exactly as I was—with all my shame, all my stuff, all my history. He had an unbounded, unconditional love for me.

I knew I still had broken parts inside me, but I reasoned, "If he's good, I'm good." If I'm honest, I didn't want to have to deal with the past anymore. That was then, this is now. I didn't want or need to go back there and touch the past.

Or did I?

I was living with a duality of bliss combined with unreconciled pain and shame from years past. I was sure all the love I had for David and his love for me would override the feelings

I'd tucked away. I thought I'd put them in a place where they couldn't interfere with all that was in front of me. But as I said before, the past is always near, and it's something no one can outrun.

When the Past Interferes with the Present

Even when we are technically out of a relationship, it doesn't mean that we have moved beyond the relationship psychologically. And if the person with whom we had a toxic relationship also shares custody of our kids, we're going to be involved with that person for years. But even if we never lay our eyes upon that toxic individual again, there is still a possibility that that past relationship will interfere with our ability to engage fully with our life at present.

In my work on narcissism, I call this the "double curse" of dating a narcissist. The first curse is the drama and sometimes abuse in the relationship itself, but even after the relationship ends, there's often a period where you get stuck trying to make sense of the past. *Why was I so*

dumb that I fell in love with this person? Why didn't I get out
sooner? Why do I keep thinking about this person? Does that
mean I still have feelings for them?

Here's the reality: When we go through a period of
intense reality distortion and gaslighting, it can be desta-
bilizing. And it's going to take some time to put the pieces
back together. But sometimes during the work of healing, people mistakenly believe that this indicates that the
past relationship was special, or that they were somehow
dumb or naive for getting involved. Certainly we all grow
through life, and we may start out more naive and grow
into wisdom through our mistakes, but falling in love with
somebody who is narcissistic or otherwise toxic happens
to all sorts of highly successful, high-functioning people.
It isn't something to be ashamed of; it's something that
happens because these narcissistic individuals are preda-
tory and deceptive. They're much more practiced at lying
and manipulation, willing to do things you would never
consider doing.

So while our past relationships don't disappear psychologically the moment they disappear physically, they will
diminish in their power over time. Have compassion for

yourself and extend yourself some grace, understanding that many individuals have been trapped in similar situations. Consider giving yourself a pat on the back for getting out and saying yes to life. Just keep making forward progress, and over time the past will become more and more distant until it seems a bit like another life.

For further reflection:

- **Name what you want in a romantic partner.** Consider how you would determine if a person you were dating had these qualities. Could you look at their history or family relationships? Could you ask them directly? Do you think your friends would have a different view of them than you or your family would?

- **Notice your patterns in relationships.** If we want to develop new, healthier patterns, we can learn from our old ones. Identify your patterns. Are you attracted to a certain type of person or do you have a certain type of feeling of infatuation that grips you?

- **Move past old challenges by saying yes to life.** How can you move past some of the struggles from your past and wake up saying yes to life? Is there something you do that makes you feel joyful and engaged? Is there a way you could arrange your life where you spend more time saying yes and less time engaging in things you find uninspiring or unenlightening?

9

DOING THE WORK

*How We Keep Moving
Toward Freedom*

t was early April, after her birthday, when Eden called to tell me about her college thesis. She said she was no longer going to carry the secrets of her father, that she was going to work toward healing herself through her art. She wanted to interview me over Zoom for the video she was making for her class. After she finished the project and turned it in to her professor, she sent it to me.

As I listened, it was difficult to hear my words, sharing with her why I felt I wasn't enough for Paulo. When I watched it, I so wanted to give myself a hug. It was never about me, but I had been living for so long in this state of "I'm not good enough. I'm not worthy. I'm not valued." This recording amplified it. It included videos of Paulo, interviews with Eden's mom and Paulo's friends, and old footage of him with other women using his charm to entice them to come to his club. Eden had found the footage on YouTube on one of her father's friend's pages.

I think this video provided an opportunity for continued closure and reconciliation for Eden. I can't speak for her, but I suspect it must have positively impacted her healing journey. It accompanied her beautiful paintings in the way my podcast would accompany the album that would be birthed in my heart. Her goals were both similar to and different from mine. I think her heart's desire was to understand and make sense of these circumstances that happened firsthand by taking control and making the video. She owned the project. She wanted answers and sought them out.

WORK #1: GIVE YOURSELF PERMISSION TO SEIZE OPPORTUNITIES TO GROW

As I listened and watched myself on camera, the words I had shared—*"Why wasn't I enough?"*—hit so very hard. And as painful as it was to watch, the video gave me a deeper understanding of how layered this story was. In a way, watching it was reassuring, knowing that nothing I had experienced was made up. The truth was simply stranger than fiction.

I was so impressed by Eden's maturity and moved by her courage. I also realized this was my emotional permission slip to explore those dark places myself. In one simple phone call, she had given me my door to freedom. Now I had to take the steps to walk through it. I borrowed her courage and let the words, lyrics, feelings, anger, shame, pain, and grief pour out of me onto any device that could hold them. I had to get these feelings out. I had always utilized songwriting and the power of music to sing what couldn't be said. Everything I've ever had to deal with I had always put into song. But this one I hadn't been able to touch. I'd been protecting Eden since she was twelve. Now she no longer needed my protection. She had found how to protect herself through her honesty, art, healing, and helping others.

What an incredible young woman with tremendous insight. Eden facing her anger and pain gave me the courage to face my own.

Likewise, you will also be given opportunities to do the work of dealing with the pain of your past. Maybe a sibling invites you to an Al-Anon support group. Or you might come across an old journal that helped you to process during an earlier season of your life. Or a friend might rave about a therapist who's been so helpful to her. Keep your eyes open for the opportunities for growth and seize them as they come. The only way around is through.

Never Stop Growing

We never stop growing and learning. We are changing, the world is changing, and the past will continually reveal new secrets.

At the beginning, this process of healing can be challenging and painful, but as we shift from healing into growth, our lives can become energized. If you're focused outwardly on the world instead of wrapped up in the pain of your old relationship, you'll notice opportunities for further growth.

It might be a high school reunion or family holiday that brings up old patterns or relationships. It might be a renewed interest in a sport or art form from when you were younger but had given up. Sometimes new challenges will arise that reactivate old wounds from the past relationship. But in all these cases there's an opportunity to become more self-aware and more engaged with life.

WORK #2: DO THE WORK IN THE WAY THAT'S SUITED TO WHO YOU ARE

I wanted to feel that unbridled freedom so much that I immediately reached out to my trusted friend and cowriter, Tori Tullier. We'd made music together before, and she is the only one I knew who could ride this wave and take this journey with me. I knew she could handle my heart in the only way someone you truly trust can.

Tori didn't hesitate. She was all in. It was April and we were set to meet in Montana in August with no other goal than to get the feelings out of me in song form—no "we have to write a hit today" or "what will the world think?" Honestly, I didn't even know if the world would ever hear my songs. I just knew I had to create them. The stories had been lodged inside me like a parasite for so long. I wanted the songs to take on the story, and I didn't want that story to inhabit me anymore.

For the twelve years that I'd been scribbling notes in my journal, recording voice memos, and creating a digital folder for photographs, I'd been unknowingly preparing for the time I spent with Tori.

August in Montana was divine, with every sunrise and sunset showing off compared to the previous day. When I picked up Tori from the airport in Bozeman, I looked at her and hugged her with all the gratitude I could emit onto another person without breaking ribs. Her demeanor is so soft, kind, and observant. She met my every step with such care. We spent the next few days in my living room, in the same room where I fell in love with David. To me this is the most sacred room in our home, with the bison hide lying across the floor in front of the fireplace and the black leather couch where David and I had shared so many wonderful conversations. This was the room where we recorded the live Montana Sessions and where our holidays are celebrated. This room is our safe room, and it's where Tori and I would turn my insides out.

> Processing my grief through music was so perfectly suited for who I was.

I rented a keyboard for her from our local music store, Music Villa, since our piano was in an alternate tuning, and for the sake of simplicity, we kept everything in 440 Hz, which is a commonly recognized standard for musical pitch. We had all the time to let the magic happen. And from years of working together, from "Selfish" to "Evel Knievel" to "Hang My Hat," we knew how to find our place in each other's songwriting space. And in our living room, I met true freedom for the first time in a dozen years. I was able to expose all the places that had been swept under the rug, all the skeletons that had been so neatly crammed into the tiny closet in my mind, one held closed by a key I had hidden in my heart. I spilled out so much of my heart and soul over those next few days. Processing my grief through music was so perfectly suited for who I was and how I was wired.

But your process may look different. It will be unique to you, even if your way to process is also through music. If you're a spiritual person, it might mean practicing prayer or meditation. If you're a wordsmith, journaling may be where your freedom comes from. If you're a creative, you might find hope and healing in paint or poetry or prose. Stay open to doing good work according to the unique ways you're wired.

WORK #3: BE GENTLE WITH YOURSELF

The song we started with was titled "The Lost Years." We already had the title; the rest was all of my pain in a waltzing 6/8 time signature. My eyes welled up with tears as it came together in three minutes of heartbreak. When the line "Will I ever be happy again?" got caught in my throat, I quickly washed it down with a little tequila. Tequila was my liquid courage when I wasn't able to face it all sober. It softened my edges and allowed layers and layers of truth to make their way out of my heart and mind and find that place between three chords and the truth. Some of it we scrapped; most of it we kept.

When the room got heavy, when we needed a break after a breakthrough, we sought nature. We hiked, we sat next to the creek, we walked to the lake, we got caught in a rainstorm, and we let the double rainbows light our way. I cooked grass-fed steaks for Tori and tried to honor her presence as much as possible. She was giving me the greatest gift. She will never truly know the extent to which she has been the catalyst for giving me the space to be present, honest, and accountable to the process. I was able to see myself through with her as my partner. She helped me pull the hinges off this closet door and helped me be okay with it getting ugly before it could become beautiful. Together we honored the process of processing.

As we finished up another song, Tori suggested, "Let's go ride horses."

A perfectly and divinely timed outing. I saddled up Magic and Stanley and we made our way over to the outdoor riding ring for Tori's first ride since she was a girl. Magic was so giving and Tori so thoughtful, they found their stride quickly. Stanley and I have been through a lot together, so we watched as we rode easy beside them. After we got the horses unsaddled and prepped to go out into the August sun, Tori walked differently. She was a cowgirl now.

We made our way back to the house, celebrated her cowgirl state of mind, and toasted a great afternoon ahead on the porch that overlooked the wedding aisle David and I keep mowed as a sweet reminder of our most special day. That day, Tori and I wrote my anthem called "The Edge," my strength song, my "when you get knocked down and pushed to your personal edge, keep going; keep working on your healing and the light will come" song.

When you commit yourself to the work of healing and transformation, you're doing a brave thing. You're choosing to face pain that many ignore. Be gentle with yourself. Practice kindness toward yourself. Do the things that bring life to your soul. And maybe take a look at the person in the mirror and tell yourself you're proud to be you and you're valued and worthy.

Being Kind to Yourself as You Heal

Just like healing the body takes time, rest, and attention, so does healing the heart and soul. Healing is a natural process that happens on its own course. It will take time and can occasionally be painful in the same way recovering from a surgery can be, but it *will* happen.

Given the slow and natural process of healing, your best bet is to be gentle on yourself and go slow. You can't heal a broken heart any faster than you can heal a broken leg. And the work of healing isn't something you need to set a speed record at.

The other important reason to go slow and be kind and gentle to yourself is so you will notice the many things around you that might help you in the healing process. These might be people you meet, books, lectures, or travel. But if you're beating yourself up in the effort to heal more quickly, you're likely to miss many of those positive things around you.

Again, it's useful to think of healing a psychological wound like a physical wound. In both cases there are things you can do to facilitate the healing process. Get proper rest, take care of your health, spend time with loved ones, and surround yourself with things that nurture your mind, body, and spirit. It might also require talking to the right experts and doing the recommended tasks to support healing. In both cases, it's best to treat yourself with kindness and have patience with the process.

WORK #4: NOTICE THE GOOD THAT HAS COME

Tori and I knew we were going to finish whatever this was with the words my mother spoke to me when Paulo died: *"Only good will come of this."* We knew its importance. We knew it would set the tone of where we would go from there.

Tori sat at her keyboard and the words and melodies came from her as if God were speaking in the room. "Only Good Will Come of This" was the last song we wrote. When we finished, we had eight songs that represented the most difficult season of my life.

As Tori headed home, David flew in. I felt so anxious, excited, and nervous for him to hear this body of work. I didn't know if it was any good, but I knew in my heart there were only two people that mattered most when hearing these songs: David and Eden.

David and I were married just outside our house by the pond with the grassy "aisle" that I had walked down. There are two red Adirondack chairs out there where we regularly watch the sunsets slip behind the endless mountain range.

I'd asked David if he would spend thirty minutes to listen to the songs Tori and I had just created—a thirty-minute run-on sentence from my heart. I wanted his honest feedback, so I asked him to pretend I wasn't his wife. He knew I wanted him to listen with fresh ears.

I sat him down and poured him a glass of tequila, neat. The songs were on my computer in chronological order. Handing him headphones, I pushed Play. He smiled, closed his eyes, and listened. He listened as my biggest fan, as my best friend. He listened hopeful and curious what this would all look like in the end.

After listening, his words settled in me so sweetly as he said, "If this hadn't happened, *we* would never have happened. You must release this music and share it with the world. It's important."

His caring confidence in this daunting task gave me the resolve I needed to take the next step, which was sharing internally with my team. The consensus was that we had something. We agreed we'd let the songs play and see what happened. In December of 2021, we met up at SIR, a rehearsal studio in Nashville, Tori on her keys, me on my guitar, and my musician family in a round so we could all make eye contact as we played the songs down. Tori and I didn't share the story behind the songs, or the magnitude of this moment, until afterward. As we weaved our way through the words and sounds, the songs did the work and left me overwhelmed with emotion and a feeling of freedom. The freedom to feel it all.

> For the first time in years, maybe in my whole life, I wasn't hiding a part of me anymore.

For the first time in years, maybe in my whole life, I wasn't hiding a part of me anymore.

The Good That Comes
with Experience

Going through a toxic relationship and coming out of it stronger is a heroic journey. And someone on a journey always returns with gifts, even if the gifts aren't enough to make up for the pain of the travel. One big gift can be a capacity for empathy. People who go through terrible experiences often gain more empathy and compassion for others who are suffering in similar ways. "The wound is the eye" is a way of saying the wounds we experience become the eyes that let us see another's suffering.

Another gift is wisdom. The process of going through a toxic relationship and having to rebuild your sense of self is challenging and forces you to look inward at your patterns and your other relationships. As a result, you'll obtain a great deal of self-knowledge and wisdom. What's nice about this is once you go through the inner work, it's harder to get rattled by other people or outside events. Your confidence will be authentic and grounded.

There are other gifts that can arise, but one I want to leave you with is gratitude. There is a deep sense of gratitude that comes from experiencing and acknowledging positive growth.

WORK #5: BE WILLING TO FEEL THE FEELS, BE WILLING TO FEEL IT ALL

After the recordings were mixed, I received them in my email. It was Christmas Eve morning, and I was sitting alone in front of our fireplace on the bison hide David had received as a wedding gift from my stepdad, Doug. This room is where we'd spent hundreds of hours together. And it's where Tori and I had written the songs that would change everything.

I sat there with my headphones on, fire blazing, and heart open, unsure of what I was about to hear. "The Lost Years" cracked me wide open, and I wept until the very last song. For me it was a complete release. It was my freedom, start to finish, packed into thirty minutes. I'd say this was the most defining moment of my life. The untold stories of so many years hidden away. Hidden behind my smiles and we-can-get-through-anything motto. What would come next? Would we share this with the world? Was it good enough? Was the story too personal? What would Eden think? And was I strong enough to walk the emotional line?

I kept many journals growing up. But the fear of someone reading my innermost thoughts eventually forced me to give it up—until that year when we would record. When David and I flew back home to Nashville, I began to write it all out: my fears, my observations, my insecurities.

Next up I would be sharing the songs with Eden to see how she felt about me presenting them to the world. Would it bring healing and closure for us? It was the most nervous I had been in a very long time. When I sent her the links, I was filled with anxiety.

Five hours later, I couldn't stand the suspense. I texted Eden.

"Did you have a chance to listen?" I queried.

The two minutes it took her to respond felt like an eternity.

"I'm feeling a lot of things."

Her response terrified me.

"Some tears too," she added.

"Me too."

Later, when we spoke on the phone, she admitted, "I don't understand why you weren't more angry."

She underscored, "You're not angry enough."

I understood what she was saying.

"Oh honey," I assured her, "I've been angry for so long."

Eden had given me permission to go to all the hard places and not worry about sparing her feelings. Who was this incredibly mature woman whom I had been sure needed my protection? She was a little girl who had lost her dad and was forced to grow up quickly. In awe of her, and knowing she was okay, I pressed on. I had worked so hard to avoid my feelings, but Eden had been brave to face hers. She inspired me. She still inspires me every day.

If you've avoided feeling what you feel—whether it's shame, remorse, guilt, anger, or anything else—I understand why. But I can testify that doing the work and acknowledging the feelings is the most life-giving path to experiencing real, true, authentic healing. And I believe you can get there too. Just like I borrowed courage from Eden, mine is yours for the taking.

Feel the Feelings

It's natural to want to avoid negative feelings following a bad relationship. At times, being able to overcome those feelings and get on with your life and back to work is of primary importance. If you have people depending on you, falling apart isn't an option. But over time you will see major psychological benefits from experiencing and processing those feelings.

We need to feel safe in order to express ourselves and our feelings. Going to a psychologist or psychotherapist is designed to provide a safe and supportive container for expressing painful emotions. Support groups are similar. And painful emotions can also be channeled in healthier ways.

Two of the healthiest places to channel painful emotions are creative pursuits and humor. Music, art, and sports stimulate the creative mind. The act of *sublimation* is when you "transform negative impulses into behaviors that are not only less damaging but sometimes productive in nature."[7] These avenues allow you to feel your emotions or express feelings in a constructive way. So much great art is channeled by deep pain, often from the end of relationships. You hear this in the blues, gospel, and old folk songs, from Bob Dylan's *Blood on the Tracks* to Taylor Swift's legendary breakup songs.

WORK #6: BE BRAVE

Although I'd completed my album, my work was not done.

I flew to LA the week before heading into the studio to

record the studio album with Paul Moak in Nashville. I wanted it to be fresh and planned on smoothing any rough edges before going into what seemed like a daunting task.

I'd made plans to meet with a woman who'd known Paulo in the days leading up to his tragic death. I pulled over a block away from the coffee shop so she wouldn't see me collecting myself before confronting her with her own words, which I had found in an email. It had been thirteen years since I'd read it, but now I had the desire to meet the truth face-to-face. She was wearing her yoga clothes; I was wearing my emotional armor.

We began with polite niceties. I didn't let on that I had evidence confirming they had been more than friends, because my friend had shared it with me even though she had asked him not to. I offered her some prompts to give her the opportunity to come clean, but she didn't. When I finally let her know I had reason to believe they'd had a relationship, she denied it—kind of. She admitted they'd gone out to dinner at a fancy restaurant and that they'd kissed.

"But," she insisted, "it was just a kiss."

What kind of horseshit is this?

None of her denials were adding up. She knew way more than she should have about Eden and me. She knew that Paulo had taken an engagement ring on our trip to Bora Bora to propose, but that he'd gotten scared. *Why would she know this? And why didn't I?*

The words she shared stung, and I prayed that neither my eyes nor my body language would give me away. I don't know if she thought sharing what she did would make it less painful. It was *all* painful. But the only way I could heal the pain was with the truth.

I left with more of what I already knew. The time with her took me back to the initial days after his death when I learned everything with him had been a lie. My stomach was in knots and reliving it with this new understanding tasted bitter in my mouth.

The following day I met with Todd, who owned the airplane Paulo had been flying when he crashed. We actually sat in the cockpit of his airplane, one similar to the plane Paulo had been flying. Paulo had always acted like he owned it, but the truth came out after his death. I'd been led to believe the plane might have been tampered with, but I needed to hear the truth from Todd. Todd told me the investigation into the crash proved it had been the result of pilot error. Confident he was telling the truth, it was the first time in thirteen years I could let go of all the unsubstantiated theories about what had happened.

The more I learned, the more I questioned. The more I questioned, the more I realized how I hadn't yet had an honest conversation with myself about my level of trauma. I thought I had brushed it off, only to find I had pushed it into the deepest part of my psyche. I was alone in the hell of it all. But as

I drove past our old rental house in the Pacific Palisades and past Eden's school, I felt like I was exactly where I was supposed to be. I thought of the years I'd allowed all this to reside inside me—so much deceit, so much smiling through layers of shame. The freedom with the songs was one thing, but sitting in the cockpit of a similar red Marchetti, understanding and accepting for the first time that the accident was truly caused by pilot error, and that there had been no conspiracy, took my breath. I put my hand on the wing and held it there, steadying myself. I wanted to throw up, but I didn't want to leave. I hadn't seen a plane like this since the night of the crash. Such a beautiful airplane, that color of red you think of when you think of red Corvettes or that perfect red lipstick. It was in pristine condition, without any scars.

The Positive Future

When you do the work of recovering and healing from a toxic relationship, you benefit personally, but so do people around you. You become more empathetic and grateful. Your life is more stable and you're able to think about other people because you're not caught up in your own drama.

Your relationships with your own family and friends will improve. You're simply a happier, more stable, more energetic, and more grounded person. Other people will respond to that. Instead of talking about Mr. Wrong during your hair appointment, you're talking about something to look forward to for the future. This helps everything around you to start moving in a positive direction. The only people who will push back on your growth are people who you might want to limit time with.

And with creative individuals, the process of healing will naturally lead to stories about the process. They will discuss it in support groups to help others who aren't quite as far along on the journey. They will make movies, paint paintings, or write songs that allow others who have had similar experiences to know they aren't alone and that there is a path forward. And maybe by working through their own negative psychological patterns, every future relationship they touch will be better off. You're not just helping yourself when you heal; you're helping everybody close to you, especially the ones who depend on you.

For further reflection:

- **Invest your emotional energy well.** Do you write, journal, or express your emotions in art or music? Do you express your emotions more physically through athletics such as dance or yoga?

- **Be kind to yourself.** If you are tough on yourself, do you think that is helping you grow? What might it look like to be a little easier on yourself? How could you practice more self-compassion?

- **Welcome the feelings you hide.** Pay attention to the feelings you don't ever dare let out. If you have hidden feelings, is there someplace safe where you think you could express them, even if just a little bit? Therapy can be a good place for this, or maybe a journal entry or in writing a poem. Identify opportunities you feel are safe to experiment with some of the feelings you're keeping bottled up.

10

WE ALL HAVE
A STORY

How We Move On with Others

All of us who'd worked together to produce our album, *On the Edge*, were working toward its release. Photoshoots, videos, and holding our breath to see what kind of national press would come on board for the release. The story—*my* story of being in a toxic relationship—was still so new for mass consumption that it wasn't ready for prime-time, late-night, or daytime TV. But then I got a "God wink."

A God wink—a term coined by author Squire Rushnell—is like a divine message to tell you you're on the right path. If there were one place in the world I could have chosen to perform on the night of my release, it would be the Grand Ole Opry.

Well, they reached out.

And when they said, "We want Stephanie here on Friday night for her release," I cried—screaming, proud, humble, emotional, ugly tears. The Opry is the greatest stage, and this would mark my twelfth performance there. Tori had never played there before, so I asked her if she would join me.

FORWARD MOTION #1: WE MOVE ON WHEN OUR STORY TOUCHES THE LIVES OF OTHERS

In the week leading up to the release, I reached out to a few of Paulo's friends. I wanted to share the music with them, to let them know it was coming, and also to ask some hard-hitting questions.

Paulo's friend Greg had been present for a lot of interesting moments in my life with Paulo, including the New Year's Eve when Paulo gave me drugs.

I texted Greg. "Hey! It's been a really long time. I wrote an album about what happened with Paulo all those years ago. Can we get on the phone?"

Largely, Greg had little recollection of this time. I'm sure, like for many of Paulo's friends, it was easier to relive the great memories amid such tragedy. I'd wanted to know what drugs Paulo had given me, but Greg didn't recall. When I asked if he'd seen Paulo with other women, he denied it. I thanked him for his time and let him know I'd send him a link to the album.

But a few days after our meeting, Greg followed up with a text.

"I listened to the album last night. It must have been cathartic for you."

Then he admitted, "I only remember one other girl, and that was at the very end."

Then, as if making excuses for Paulo, he offered, "When it came to marrying you, he was struggling with the idea of being domesticated."

Some of what I learned when I reached out to Paulo's friends stung because it was all true. And sometimes I think maybe I wanted someone to call me out as a liar, that I had fabricated this whole thing.

Maybe I had made this all up in my head, I'd reason in the days leading up to the album release. *Should I pull the album?* That week I was sick to my stomach. *What was I thinking? Will this insane story really help people?*

And then Friday came, the album went live, and the weight of those last thirteen years started to peel away as messages flooded my inboxes on every platform. I wasn't alone; my story wasn't unique. It broke my heart to hear from so many hurting people, but it also fortified my resolve to share more. Now I know that truth and vulnerability is what sets us free—not smiling through our internal or external pain and shame.

The sharing of my story will live on beyond me, and it's about as public as it gets! But guess what? You get to decide how you do or don't share your story. That's your choice. But what I can tell you is there's power when you're willing to let your story touch the lives of others. When others hear it and witness your redemption, they begin to see what's possible. So I do hope you'll consider how your story might be a gift to others in whatever shape that takes for you.

Sharing Our Stories

There are powerful benefits to sharing stories. Psychologically speaking, when we reveal parts of ourselves that have been hidden or trapped, it feels freeing, even cathartic. We no longer need to constantly defend against the truth or make excuses. We can move beyond the story. Eventually, there will be a new story to tell, and hopefully it will be less pain-filled and more love-filled.

But there are also some good reasons why people don't want to share their stories. When you're telling your story, you aren't the only character in it. Your story might involve your family or other loved ones, coworkers, and colleagues, even organizations you belong to. Ethically, there's nothing wrong with telling your story, but it gets more challenging when you tell other people's stories without their knowledge or consent.

There are a couple of good approaches for handling this. First, you can reach out to those people from your past and ask them if they mind being in the story. You can even ask for their personal impressions that might help fill out your story. You can also disguise individuals, so they don't become public figures. People who know you might have some ideas who you're talking about, but your general listeners or audience won't. The great psychologist Sigmund Freud always gave pseudonyms when writing about his patients to keep their identity protected.

When it comes to stories about family that involves some dirty laundry, my suggestion is to have the hard conversations with family members before making everything public. It's never easy, but if people know what's coming, they can prepare themselves and not get blindsided.

FORWARD MOTION #2: WE MOVE ON WHEN WE EMBRACE OUR UNIQUE PURPOSE

Music is so powerful. When I performed "The Lost Years" in the Opry Circle, I also shared the story. The room gasped. Then I invited Tori out and she and I played "Only Good Will Come of This," just us two on the grand ole stage. I was so proud, not only of the intense work we did together, the songs we created and believed in together, but for her to feel the magnitude of that stage, to introduce her to the world on that stage, and to say to her after her piano solo, "Hey, Tori, you're at the Grand Ole Opry!"

The crew who showed up to support us was amazing. David was there, along with Carli and Christine, who run my company. My best friend, Celine, and her fiancé, Chris, were there. Tori's mom and her boyfriend were there. My friend Amy brought her parents. And many other amazing friends were there too.

What a gift and treasure it was. Although Eden wasn't able

to make it to the event, I got to talk to her from the stage in hopes she might be listening to the Opry radio. I lost it then. I love her so. If floating on musical clouds is possible, that's what we were doing. And the ether that followed the next few days was intensified with every story shared from strangers and friends alike.

We followed up with a music video of "The Lost Years" that premiered in Times Square with CMT. We flew up to New York for the day and it was magic. Next, we released our short film with *People* magazine, sharing the snapshots of the story in a very PG-rated version of the entire album.

> If floating on musical clouds is possible, that's what we were doing.

As I have been learning, discovering, and then discovering more, this story doesn't end here. It's only the beginning. And with the amount of healing the songs, the journaling, and the writing have elicited, I feel a sense of purpose now like never before.

What about you? What will embracing a new sense of purpose look like for you? It may simply mean that you live with a renewed sense of courage and transparency. Or you may choose to shepherd others who are facing what you once faced. You are the one who gets to choose how you will steward or share all that you've experienced.

Our Stories and Our Purpose

Our stories are part of who we are, and sharing those stories is a way of communicating our experience to a wider audience. When we tell our personal story, it becomes a shared one. Storytelling is central to the experience of being human. Humans have gathered around campfires for millennia sharing stories that were dramatic, scary, exciting, and humorous.

Some people are so good at storytelling that it becomes their profession or purpose in life. The great poets and bards of old sang stories about great heroes before we had access to books. These bards would wander the world reciting stories in exchange for food or acclaim. Eventually these stories were written down and became works such as *The Odyssey*, the Bible, folk music, and poetry. The best stories are individual to us but reflect a common theme among people. Your heartbreak, for example, might be extremely personal, but when you share it with other people, it allows them to reexperience and process their own heartbreak in a new and hopefully healthier way.

FORWARD MOTION #3: WE MOVE
ON WHEN WE FORGIVE

On the fourteenth anniversary of Paulo's death, I realized I still hadn't forgiven him.

At the time, I was in Nashville, going through my regular morning routine of meditation and prayers that I had learned from Vishen Lakhiani's book, *The 6 Phase Meditation Method*. The daily rhythm had six phases: compassion, gratitude, forgiveness, vision for my life, vision for the day, and prayer. I rolled through the first two, but when I got to the third, forgiveness, I was suddenly awestruck. The realization that I had never forgiven Paulo hit me.

I'm a big believer that forgiveness doesn't have anything to do with the other person saying they're sorry or repenting. I believe it has everything to do with us. And it's the thing that can finally give us our lives back.

Overwhelmed with emotion, I felt the sting of unforgiveness viscerally. And when I decided I never wanted to feel that way again, I chose to film my expression of forgiveness. Maybe I'd share it with Eden.

Wearing my black turtleneck, speaking directly to the camera, I filmed myself forgiving Paulo.

After I hit Stop, I sent it to my team, Carli and Christine, for their input.

"Is this for me and Eden?" I asked them. "Or is it for the world?"

"Could other people benefit, or is it just ego?" I added. "If it serves others, it's worth sharing."

"If you're willing, I think this will help a lot of people," they both responded.

Eden, really the only audience who mattered to me, saw it on socials. Texting me, she let me know she was happy I'd forgiven her dad.

And me? I felt lighter. I felt relieved. And I felt like maybe this would give others a chance more quickly to forgive someone who hurt them after seeing me release this heavy burden. It's so hard on our bodies to carry that much pain. Our bodies remember it all.

It was hard but healing.

I also forgave the Prince.

And myself.

I am free.

Forgiveness

When someone betrays us, the natural response might be either to avoid that person or to seek revenge. This is normal but can also be a hard way to live. You can become consumed with thoughts of the individual who betrayed you. While it may feel momentarily satisfying, revenge is rarely enough for healing.

When you forgive someone, it doesn't mean making excuses for their behavior or agreeing that what they did wasn't harmful. And it certainly doesn't mean forgetting what they did, reestablishing a relationship, or even trusting them again. Instead, forgiveness means dropping your resentment or negativity toward the person, letting go of your ill will for the betrayal, and moving forward in your life without the psychological baggage of the betrayal.

Through forgiveness, you become free of the haunting thoughts about this person and start to see them more as someone who is perhaps malicious but also broken.

More importantly, you don't necessarily forgive someone for *their* benefit. You forgive them for your own benefit. It's impossible to go back in time and undo what was done, but it *is* possible to stop carrying the pain, resentment, and hostility you feel toward the person. And without carrying that pain, you will feel much freer and more available to say yes to your future.

For further reflection:

- **Practice forgiveness.** Have you ever forgiven someone who hurt you? How did you feel afterward? Did you tell them you forgave them, or did you decide to keep it to yourself? If you did share it with them, what was that experience like?

- **Take responsibility for your wrongs.** Sometimes we're the wrongdoers, accidental or otherwise. Have you ever received the benefit of someone else's forgiveness? How, if at all, did it change your behavior moving forward?

- **Notice, and own, your temptation to blame.** Even if you're in an otherwise healthy relationship, sometimes small resentments show up. Maybe your partner didn't take out the trash like they said they would, or maybe they overspent on the grocery budget. Who in your life have you not forgiven yet? What might it be like for you to do the work to forgive them? What steps might you take to move in that direction?

AFTERWORD

Why *do* we stay?

I'm still doing the work to understand why I stayed—in more than one relationship. And I'm grateful for how far I've come on this journey.

I learned many of these lessons later in life than I wish I had. The lost years are gone. But today my time is more precious to me than ever before. I don't get lost in the things I can't control anymore.

Today, I trust my gut. If it feels right, I press in. If it doesn't, I walk away. I welcome quiet. The quiet is where my thoughts get to make themselves known. I don't push them away anymore; I invite them to say what they have to say, and to stay awhile.

Over the course of these last few years, I've learned to love myself. I know it sounds cliché, but here's the truth I'm living: I don't put myself down anymore. I don't swim in shame. I look in the mirror in the worst lighting after no sleep and find something nice to say about myself. I look back on everyone who has come in and out of the saloon doors of my life with a lot more grace and understanding.

What if true love is first and foremost about truly loving yourself? Then everyone who loves you after that is gravy. No, *better* than gravy: whipped cream topping, perfectly chilled, topped with shredded dark chocolate and a few fresh, ripe raspberries.

I'm excited for David to get the best of me now, and for me to get to experience her too.

My life's purpose is to share my stories so that more light will shine on you. And I want you to hear that just as my story matters, *your* story matters. Your courage matters. Your vulnerability matters. *You* matter.

Beloved, if you are in a toxic relationship, don't stay. You deserve to be emotionally and physically safe. You deserve to be loved well.

Wherever you are on this journey today, I am cheering you on as you take your next step toward freedom. I am always here, with courage for you to borrow and a heart to listen.

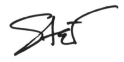

ACKNOWLEDGMENTS

This body of work was made possible because of the support around me. I'd like to acknowledge and thank the many extraordinary people along this journey. (I am a wordy woman, so if you don't see your name, I had to use invisible ink continued on to the next page!)

God, thank You for never leaving me, even when I was sure I knew better. Thank You for being the greatest conductor of my life symphony. Thank You for righting and lighting my path in the darkest, most devastating hours.

My most precious family, what a gift you are. I am in awe of each one of you and your unwavering belief in me and our family. Dad, I am a little you. Mom, just like you said, "only good." Loretta, we did it. Doug, thank you for loving me like your own.

Husband, your patience, love, and devotion are unmatched. Thank you for seeing all my edges and sides as catalysts toward greatness and never as deterrents. Thank you for loving me as I found my personal freedom through this self-discovery process. (I am more fun now, yes?!)

Thank you, Sara and Andrew, my stepkids, for wanting the world for me. I love you both with every fiber of my being.

Eden, you are my heart, my little moon. You might not be my biological daughter, but I will always love you like you are. I cherish you and thank you for your courage. I borrow it every day.

Carli Kane and Christine D'Ancona of Big Sky Music Group, my team, my confidants. This is ours to share with the world. Thank you for meeting me in every moment and emotion with such grace, integrity, character, and determination, to see me through every revelation and every note.

Tori Tullier, all those years ago I never could've imagined where our stories and songs would take us. Here's to many more hummingbird, double-rainbow-filled Montana skies. You have provided me with a safe passage through song, and I will never forget that.

John Zarling, thank you for taking a great chance on me and my story and sharing it with our HarperCollins family. Michael Aulisio, Kara Mannix, Bonnie Honeycutt, Margot Starbuck, Robin Richardson, and the entire staff, thank you for believing in me and my purpose, elevating my story, and growing its wings beyond my wildest vision.

Thank you, Chase Reynolds Ewald, Ken Amorosano with *COWGIRL* magazine, and Edyie Bryant and the entire Wrangler team. Our cover story was the spark that led me to sharing my whole story.

Dr. Scott Barry Kaufman, thank you for asking me "what I was drinking about" that fateful night that led us to a friendship and ultimately bringing Dr. Keith Campbell into my heart and world.

Keith, I will never forget our first conversation and the honesty and comfort your words brought me. Thank you for lending your heart, wisdom, and professional perspective into my life experience. I know the impact on the world will be great.

GLOSSARY

This glossary contains a variety of words and phrases related to relationships, some of which have been discussed in this book.

ABUSE: An intentional effort by a partner to cause harm. Abuse can be physical, such as striking a partner, but it can also be emotional with the goal of causing emotional suffering or control.

ATTACHMENT STYLE: In infancy and early childhood, people learn how relationships work through their relationships with their parents or other caregivers. As the child grows into an adult, these early attachment experiences develop into models or beliefs about how relationships work. (See also *Insecure Attachment Style* and *Secure Attachment Style*.)

CODEPENDENCY: A form of dysfunctional caregiving relationship where one partner in the relationship sacrifices themselves to care for the other partner. The cared-for partner might be engaged in self-destructive behaviors, like drug or alcohol use or gambling disorders. Codependency does not refer to taking care of a sick or injured spouse in a healthy way.

COGNITIVE DISSONANCE: The uncomfortable psychological state that arises when our beliefs and our behaviors do not line up. For example, if we think our partner is a loving, caring person and our partner is abusive to us, this can result in a state of psychological dissonance. This psychological dissonance can be resolved by changing your beliefs about the partner—for example, by acknowledging they are abusive or by leaving the relationship—or in a less healthy way by making excuses for the partner's behavior and not being honest with yourself about their abusiveness.

DARK TRIAD: The dark triad is a group of three psychological traits that are each related to interpersonal antagonism or meanness. These three traits that make up the dark triad are narcissism, psychopathy, and Machiavellianism.

DEFENSE MECHANISMS: Psychological structures that keep threatening information away from our awareness. Defense mechanisms include *denial* or pretending something didn't happen; *projection* or placing the negative beliefs or emotions onto someone else; or *intellectualization,* where we think rationally about a painful issue but don't allow ourselves to experience the painful emotions.

EGO SHOCK: A brief "freezing" of consciousness, psychological numbness, and confusion that can accompany major blows to self-esteem. These blows can include failure, romantic rejection, or humiliation.

GAME-PLAYING / MIND GAMES: Displaying commitment to the relationship at times and then displaying disinterest at other times. For example, a game-playing partner might talk about marriage and commitment one day and the next day say, "Oh, I was just joking about that." A partner who is game-playing often leaves their partner feeling uncertain and powerless.

GASLIGHTING: A strategy for psychologically manipulating another person into thinking they are going crazy or losing touch with reality. The term *gaslighting* comes from an old movie where the protagonist would turn the lights down in the house but deny doing so (along with other tricks) to make his wife think she was going insane. It's important to have contact with reality to resist gaslighting. For example, having close friends or a therapist you trust to talk with.

GROOMING: A long-term strategy to gain trust and physical and emotional intimacy through a series of incremental steps that start out more casual and transparent and then become more secretive and intimate.

INSECURE ATTACHMENT STYLE: A more unstable home or tragedy growing up can lead to less trust and stability in relationships.

LOVE BOMBING: A large amount of positive attention and praise given to a potential romantic partner who is overwhelmed by the affection and falls under the spell of the love bomber. After commitment is established, the love bombing diminishes and is replaced with efforts to control.

MANIPULATION (ALSO EXPLOITATION): *Manipulation* and *exploitation* are terms used to describe controlling someone's thoughts, feelings, or behaviors in underhanded or devious ways.

NARCISSISM: A personality trait describing an inflated sense of oneself along with a relative lack of compassion or empathy for other people. Narcissists can manipulate and exploit others and have a powerful craving for attention and admiration.

NARCISSISTIC PERSONALITY DISORDER (NPD): The psychiatric personality disorder associated with extreme narcissism. NPD is a combination of grandiose self-views, a lack of empathy for others, and a need for positive attention and admiration. Importantly, NPD leads to significant impairment in the individual's love and work lives.

PSYCHOPATHY: A combination of antagonism, hostility, self-centeredness, and impulsivity. Psychopathy can be a personality trait, but at the extremes, psychopathy can be a personality disorder that is sometimes linked to criminality.

REPETITION COMPULSION: This behavior involves repeating painful situations that occurred in the past. It's a way to ease tension from physical or emotional trauma, but it doesn't always work that way. This unconscious "trauma reenactment" can include any experience where you feel overwhelmed with hopelessness or fear.

SECURE ATTACHMENT STYLE: With healthy parents and a loving home, you typically see a secure attachment style that includes high trust in others.

SOCIOPATH: Someone who has an antagonistic and impulsive personality style that makes it hard to engage in the social world in a healthy way. Sociopathic behavior often leads to criminality. The terms *sociopath* and *psychopath* are often used interchangeably, although a sociopath is more of a social term and a psychopath is more of a psychological term.

TOXIC RELATIONSHIP: A relationship between two people who don't relate to each other in healthy ways and have more conflict than is typical or necessary. One person exploits, distorts, or minimizes the perspective and experience of the other person. In this kind of relationship, neither partner is growing or flourishing. Instead, you see hostility, anxiety, uncertainty, victimization, and abuse.

TRAUMA: An intense negative experience that leaves a lasting psychological impact. Trauma can range from the extreme levels of military combat and sexual assault to highly challenging emotional trauma.

TRAUMA BONDING: A pattern of abuse from an individual that is broken up by efforts at connection. Over time, this can lead to an emotional bond being formed with the abusive partner.

NOTES

1. Stephanie Quayle, "Charmed," *On the Edge*, Big Sky Music Group, 2022.
2. Sarah Barkley, "What Is Repetition Compulsion?" PsychCentral, updated September 16, 2022, https:// psychcentral.com/blog/repetition-compulsion-why-do -we-repeat-the-past.
3. Kirsten Weir, "Nurtured by Nature," *Monitor on Psychology* 51, no. 3 (April/May 2020): 50, https://www .apa.org/monitor/2020/04/nurtured-nature.
4. Anahad O'Connor, "How Food May Improve Your Mood," *New York Times*, updated December 21, 2021, https:// www.nytimes.com/2021/05/06/well/eat/mental-health -food.html
5. Leo Galland, "The Gut Microbiome and the Brain," *Journal of Medicinal Food* 17, no. 12 (December 2014): 1261–1272, https://doi.org/10.1089/jmf.2014.7000.
6. Zara Abrams, "The Case for Kindness," American Psychological Association, August 2021, https://www.apa .org/news/apa/kindness-mental-health.
7. Kendra Cherry, "What Is Sublimation in Psychology?" Verywell Mind, updated December 14, 2022, https://www .verywellmind.com/what-is-sublimation-in-psychology -4172222.

ABOUT THE AUTHORS

Stephanie Quayle is a Nashville recording artist who tours the world with her music and an entrepreneur with her own record label, Big Sky Music Group. *Rolling Stone* Country called her "an artist you need to know," *CMT* named her as part of its "Next Women of Country" franchise, and she's appeared on popular programs like *The Kelly Clarkson Show* and *The Ellen DeGeneres Show*. As an indie artist with two Billboard charted singles, "Selfish" and "Whatcha Drinkin 'Bout," she has repeatedly performed at CMA Fest and the Grand Ole Opry. The Montana native has teamed up with recognizable brands like Wrangler, Harley-Davidson, Bass Pro Shops, Montana Silversmiths, as well as Lucchese Bootmaker in the creation of her exclusive boot line. Quayle's latest album *On the Edge* chronicles her personal experience in a toxic relationship and the healing she's gone through since—inspiring others and redefining her future.